THE OLD AGE CHALLENGE TO THE BIOMEDICAL MODEL:
PARADIGM STRAIN AND HEALTH POLICY

Charles F. Longino, Jr.
Wake Forest University, North Carolina

and

John W. Murphy
University of Miami, Coral Gables

Jon Hendricks, Editor
SOCIETY AND AGING SERIES

Baywood Publishing Company, Inc.
Amityville, New York

Library of Congress Catalog card Number: 94-30642
ISBN: 0-89503-165-5 (cloth)
ISBN: 0-89503-167-1 (Paper)

Library of Congress Cataloging-in-Publication Data

Longino, Charles F., 1938-
    The old age challenge to the biomedical model : paradigm strain
and health policy / Charles F. Longino, Jr. and John W. Murphy.
      p. cm. - - (Society and aging series)
    Includes bibliographical references and index.
    ISBN 0-89503-165-5 (cloth). - - ISBN 0-89503-167-1 (pbk.)
    1. Medical policy- -United States. 2. Medical care- -United States-
-Forecasting. 3. Aged- -Medical care- -United States. I. Murphy,
John W. II. Title. III. Series: Society and aging.
    [DNLM: 1. Health Policy- -United States. 2. Aged. 3. Delivery of
Health Care- -organization & administration- -United States. WT 30
L855 1995]
RA395.A3L67 1995
362.1'0973- -dc20
DNLM/DLC
for Library of Congress   94-30642
                                          CIP

For Loyce

FOREWORD

At least since the mid-nineteenth century, scientific discussions of aging have shunned existential uncertainties and social values, narrowing their focus to presumably answerable questions studied with rigorous methods. In his *Clinical Lectures on the Diseases of Old Age* (1861), the French physician Jean Charcot endorsed the idea that science would someday attain "complete knowledge" of the normal man and of "all the secrets of the pathological condition." Charcot's colleague Claude Bernard went further: "A living organism is nothing but a wonderful machine," wrote Bernard in his classic *An Introduction to the Study of Experimental Medicine* (1865). "We know absolutely nothing about the essence . . . of life; but we shall nevertheless regulate vital phenomena as soon as we know enough of their necessary conditions."

In the late nineteenth century, the new experimental methodology began influencing the biomedical study of aging. Laboratory scientists discarded older theories based on the exhaustion of some vital element (e.g., heat, moisture, energy) and focused their attention on progressively narrower, empirically observable changes taking place in organs, tissues, and cells. The founders of modern gerontology and geriatrics—men like Elie Metchnikoff and I. L. Nascher—believed it was possible to discover immutable laws of normality and pathology as applied to senescence. They assumed that these laws—divorced from their cultural and social contexts—would yield authoritative knowledge about aging. Medicine would supply the therapeutic agents to combat disease and restore healthy normality.

A century later, the rise of chronic illness in our aging society has demolished the dreams of a disease-free old age and revealed that the line between the normal and the pathological is not always clear and distinct. Yet medical practice and research remain largely modeled on acute disease. Meanwhile, the exclusive claims and methods of modern science have yielded to awareness of multiple kinds of knowledge and ways of knowing. Yet gerontological research and practice remain dominated by the modern scientific world view of its founders. In *The Old Age Challenge to the Biomedical Model: Paradigm Strain and Health Policy*, Charles F. Longino, Jr. and John W. Murphy challenge this state of affairs. "The key point in this book," they write, "is that a complete philosophical shift will be necessay if chronicity is to be dealt with adequately."

Longino and Murphy's major contribution lies in joining certain strands of postmodern thinking to a critique of acute-care medicine and its disempowering professional claims to expert knowledge. Postmodern theorists (e.g., Foucault, Deleuze and Guattari, Lyotard, and Rorty) generally reject a major premise of modern science and philosophy—that theory mirrors reality, that objective human knowledge provides an untainted Archimedean point from which see the world correctly and completely. Instead they argue that there is no epistemologically privileged place to stand apart from the objects one studies. Scientists never achieve a pure picture of reality, only particular renditions framed by interested observers in particular circumstances.

The Old Age Challenge to the Biomedical Model attempts to drive home the ethical and political implications of these ideas in the arenas of chronic illness and health policy. The realization that all knowledge is partial and humanly situated has radically democratic implications. Following Harry R. Moody and others who have written about the ethics of aging, Longino and Murphy argue that technical expertise (presumed to be methodologically rigorous and value-free) should be replaced by Habermas's notion of "communicative competence," which, for example, would allow definitions of risk, health, and illness to be shaped by a dialogue between physician and patient.

Longino and Murphy would extend the democratization of knowledge beyond the doctor/patient relationship to health policy. In the current era of health care reform, they believe that uncritical acceptance of the marketplace and technical expertise have overshadowed the importance of public participation in health care. An informed and active citizenry, increased local control, an emphasis on interpretative methodologies and context-based information, and collective resource allocation—these are among the authors' key recommendations for achieving a more socially responsive health care system better equipped to handle the challenge of chronic illness. While Longino and

Murphy's ideals will seem "unrealistic" to many, the demographic and the democratic nature of chronic illness in the postmodern era may well be on their side.

Thomas R. Cole, Director
Institute for the Medical Humanities
University of Texas Medical Branch at Galveston

ACKNOWLEDGMENTS

There are a list of people that we wish to thank. Phil Perricone provided the occasion to think hard and long about the philosophy of medicine due to a new course assignment. The University of Miami payed for John Murphy to visit Wake Forest University to give three talks, to meet the Bell brothers, and to conspire about this book. Joe Hendricks encouraged us to consider writing a book in Baywood's Society and Aging Series. Mildred Seltzer asked us to summarize parts of our argument into a chapter of a future-looking book that she was editing. The dauntless students in the Social Psychology of Health and Illness course at Wake Forest listened endlessly and responded to many of the arguments of the book as the early drafts appeared. The comments and other reactions, especially those from Melanie Angiollio, Crystal Bowie, Edward Chung, Jessica Davey, Marlene Mancuso, Peter Milner, Catherine Peacock, Ben Selan, Chad Simpson, Shannon Stokes, and Hillary Theakston were helpful and appreciated. Mark Smith, a postdoctoral fellow in the department of internal medicine and gerontology at the Bowman Gray School of Medicine, contributed ideas on long term care and epidemiological research. Pam Teaster from Virginia Tech., and David Frankford from Rutgers responded helpfully to an early draft of the manuscript. Carol Corum entered several chapters and revisions of hand written script onto disk and kept track of which was the latest revision of a continuously evolving manuscript. Her endurance and good spirit made the process as pleasant as it could be. Tom Cole, Director of the Institute for the Medical Humanities at the University of Texas Medical Branch at Galveston, generously agreed to add his two cents in a foreword. John Gregg, David Kammann, and Andrea Badillo did their share of proofing, copying, and mailing. Stella Cline was a good library sleuth, and Jennifer Sanderson and Will Corum helped with the page proofs. The production staff at Baywood performed wonderfully, especially Bobbi Olszewski who went beyond her usual duties to expedite the process. Our wives provided inspiration and forebearance, and Charles and Laura Longino listened and encouraged. To each of them we voice our gratitude.

Table of Contents

Introduction

THE BIOMEDICAL MODEL AND REDUCTIONISM

A juggernaut is driving the health care system to a predicament affording no obvious escape. On the one hand, biomedicine is sustained by a set of assumptions that guide the medical enterprise. On the other, these presuppositions are incompatible with treating chronic illness. The problem is that as the population ages, this sort of malady will become even more prevalent. As a result, the prevailing medical system may become irrelevant and rapidly outmoded.

At this time, the rise of chronicity is receiving much attention. Most persons seem to recognize that as the "baby boom" generation ages, for example, a variety of social changes will occur. But the impact on the medical system has been underestimated. Practitioners have begun to recognize that perhaps some new services will be required. These additions, however, are planned to be introduced at the periphery of the traditional medical enterprise. Little awareness seems to be present about how the philosophy that underpins biomedicine may render this approach to medical practice ineffective in the near future. The key point in this book is that a complete philosophical shift will be necessary, if chronicity is to be dealt with adequately. In other words, the core of current medicine will have to be altered, or chronic problems will be misconstrued and mistreated.

In this discussion the biomedical model is understood to have five components. These are 1) the mind and body are essentially different and medicine is restricted to considerations related to the body; 2) the body can be understood as analogous to a machine; 3) medical answers are thought to be more reliable when they are founded on basic sciences, and thus biophysical answers are preferred to all others; 4) a singular and specific cause exists for every disease, and through biomedical science each cause can be discovered and a cure provided for every illness; and 5) a patient's physiology is the proper focus of the regimen and control enacted by the physician [1]. The principal short-coming of this model is that it is too narrow to handle the complex nature of chronic medical problems. In short, the biomedical model is reductionistic.

This pronouncement is hardly new; the restrictive character of biomedicine has been debated for quite some time. Nonetheless, the overall effectiveness of biomedicine was not called into question. Indeed, most acute illnesses responded nicely to biomedical interventions, and those who criticized the biomedical model were considered to be misguided or uninformed. The precipitous increase in chronic disease that is expected, however, will likely alter this assessment. As never before, widespread chronicity may shake the foundations of biomedicine. Criticism of biomedicine may be essential if medical treatment is to have any positive effects in the near future.

A distinction has always been made between those afflictions that have a sudden onset, rage briefly, and then leave abruptly, such as most infectious diseases, and those that begin slowly and lead to gradually increasing disability. The former afflictions have been thought of as "acute" and the latter as "chronic." Before this century, there were some prevalent disabling infectious diseases, too, such as tuberculosis and syphilis, that by this distinction should be considered as chronic. Nevertheless, as Fox writes, "The phrase *chronic disease* came to be used . . . as a loose descriptor for illnesses of slow onset and long course, for which a singular and specific cause had not yet been discovered" [2, p. 23]. When advocates of biomedicine are reminded that they have not discovered a cure for cancer or diabetes, "promissory notes," such as "We're working on it," are issued to salvage the bio-medical model [3]. In this way, the inconsistency between the bio-medical model and chronicity is concealed.

The impact of acute and chronic disease on the patient is different because an acute disorder is distinct and limited, and its cause and treatment are understood. In a chronic condition, however, the whole person is tormented, and where the malady came from and where it will go is not well understood. Therefore, clear and concise cures are not readily available. As Cassell affirms, "When suffering occurs in the course of acute disease, medical understandings of the body and categories of disease seem adequate to explain why the threat to the integrity of person exists" [4, p. 48]. This is not so with a chronic disease that grinds away at the person, his or her associates and family, or even the community.

Distinctions are made in the medical community between primary, secondary, and tertiary prevention. Primary prevention pertains to the diagnosis and treatment of a disease *before it is manifest*. Inoculation and education to avoid a disease are primary strategies and are associated with public health approaches to illness, or calcium supplementation and exercise in young women to offset later postmenopausal osteoporotic bone loss.

Secondary prevention is defined as treating a disease *to prevent recurrence or progression once manifest.* For example, the earliest manifestations of arteriosclerotic heart disease can be found even in the arteries of children. Lifestyle changes to slow or even stop the progress of early heart disease are examples of secondary prevention. In terms of acute manifestation, as after a heart attack, prevention aimed at postponing a second heart attack would also fall into this category. One would expect primary and secondary prevention to expand greatly as managed care systems come to dominate the organization of clinical medicine. In the past, however, these sorts of strategies have been aimed primarily at preventing the reoccurrance of acute disease manifestations.

Tertiary prevention is aimed at *restoration of function once disease has caused dysfunction.* Nearly all rehabilitation strategies fall into this category, including the work of physical and occupational therapists.

Levels of preventive strategies should not be confused with levels of care or services. Primary care is considered to be the first encounter with a practitioner when the patient presents his or her health concerns. Secondary and tertiary care services are a matter of degree of complexity and the sophistication of technology, generally delivered by specialists and subspecialists. Ostensibly, tertiary services treat severe disorders to save the patient's life, at least in the short run; heart bypass surgery or a cancer operation are examples. As Pelletier argues, "most of the medical care given today is tertiary care . . . , care which attempts to bring about curative results, alleviate suffering, restore the maximum possible degree of function and prolong life at any cost" [5]. Tertiary care is aimed at treatment and thus tends to deal with chronic disease only after manifestation, and often in its final stages. This strategy is heroic. And, in keeping with the American national character, it embodies crises-management rather than planning. Further, tertiary care is considered to be "scientific medicine," and thus the medical profession is reluctant to invest a lot of time, effort, and money in the care associated with primary prevention, which is considered to use low-tech and less interesting forms of mediation. But as should be noted, primary prevention applies well to chronic illness. Chronicity requires that serious attention be extended to prevention and that care be broadened or made more holistic. In short, prevention, maintenance, and management must receive greater emphasis.

There is a continuing aspect of care involving maintenance and management that is especially important to older patients. This is care for persons with disabilities that result from chronic disorders, and takes the form of "long-term care." Delegated to medical social workers and nurses by the medical establishment, long-term care has tended to be devalued by the medical subspecialists. This practice is viewed only as custodial and thus unworthy of biomedicine. Hence, in the past, little attention has been given by physicians to the rehabilitative potentialities of long-term care patients. As the older population in the United States continues to grow, however, long-term care will likely come to dominate a broader version of medicine than now exists.

HOLISTIC MEDICINE AND CHRONIC ILLNESS

Other writers, such as Knowles [6], Graubard [7], and Waldovski [8] have tried to illustrate this emergence of chronic illness, but their efforts were not critical enough. These have been mostly instrumental responses that do not challenge the basic philosophy of biomedicine. An adequate response will require a shift away from the curative bias of traditional medicine, so that emphasis can be placed on the whole person. As part of this change, interaction will have to be understood to exist between the mind and body, patient and the environment, and physiology and culture. Persons, in short, must be viewed as actively involved in the promotion of health. Stated differently, they are not the passive recipients of disease agents or medical knowledge. With regard to chronicity, a social context exists that should not be ignored when formulating an intervention. A plethora of social and cultural factors should receive attention, which have minimal importance in the use of biomedicine.

Attention will have to be broadened so that holistic approaches will gain legitimacy and be used more widely, thereby breaking free of the monopoly that grants to biomedicine hegemony in all health matters. (See pp. 76-78 for definitions.) But critics should recognize that the ideology of medicine and its structure are linked. For example, legislation and organizational rules have justified the rewards and narrow focus of the medical profession. But the stress on physiology originates from the primacy that is given in the biomedical model to biological theory. As a result, the health care system is hierarchical; at the center of traditional medicine are issues of power, territoriality and exclusiveness [9, pp. 33, 47]. In feminist terms, the medical system is patriarchal. In post-modernist terms, it is dualistic. The point is that the structure of health care cannot be divorced from the philosophy of biomedicine. They are mutually reinforcing. Accordingly, changing one without the other will probably be unproductive. Yet at this juncture in the development of health care policy in the United States, this inter-play between philosophy and practice is receiving scant attention.

Scientific medicine cannot approach chronicity because of the dualis-tic way in which disease is defined. Furthermore, dualism legitimizes the hierarchical practices that are adopted to provide care. In fact, essential to the biomedical model is a dualism that rationalizes trans-forming persons into physiological objects. This same dualism, accord-ingly, plays an instrumental role in elevating medical opinions over all others, and in excluding patients from their own treatment [10, pp. 9-10].

Cassell contends that practitioners of scientific medicine are more interested in pursuing a disease than caring for a sick person. Accord-ing to the dictates of biomedicine, the person, sick or otherwise, is not the focus of inquiry, but the body of a patient. And within the body the physician seeks out a disease which is given an ontological status through classification. Stated simply, a disease is a discrete entity that can be discovered, treated, and cured.

Thus far, there are two interlocking dualistic distinctions: first, the body delimits the parameters of medical inquiry, while, second, inter-vention is restricted to disease. As might be expected, these dualistic distinctions have far reaching implications. For instance, in the diag-nostic process there are symptoms and perceptions of the patient that are considered to be subjective by the physician, and signs and observa-tions made by the physician, using today's medical technology, that are considered objective [11]. And as Cassell notes, in the scientific era of medicine "the word objective [has] come to have the connotation of real, in contrast to subjective things which are only mental and therefore unreal" [4, p. 96]. Because the body is grounded in nature and thus real, physiological indices of disease are treated as factual. Insights offered by patients, because this information is deemed subjective, are downplayed in importance. But suffering is not found in the physiology of a person. In point of fact, health and illness are human constructs. And given this insensitivity to the human condition, biomedicine has little chance of dealing productively with chronic disease. More holistic approaches are needed to deal with chronicity because relief from the suffering associated with this problem often resides outside of the body.

Good reports that chronic pain is often embedded in repressed symbolism, performance failure, and fear [12]. Chronicity, in this sense, is linked inextricably to social conditions. This is regularly the case with acute illness. But in the example of chronic disease, ignoring this relationship becomes very difficult. In a sense, chronicity exem-plifies the tie that is present between the mind and body, and the self and *Umwelt*.

Furthermore, chronic disease is dynamic rather than static. This kind of malady lies dormant as "potential"—present in a pre-clinical form—and then is finally manifested. In the end, this condition progresses to a crisis, which can at best be managed. Usually pregnancy is characterized as an either-or situation, but heart disease cannot be identified this simply. Chronic diseases operate on a continuum, one that, in some cases, can increase or decrease depending on a host of conditions. The conceptual basis of biomedicine, with its ontological demands, makes it difficult to conceptualize, assess, and predict chronic disease. In biomedicine, disease must be present physiologically or it does not exist. Talk about potential, pre-clinical status, and situational contingencies is not concise enough for scientists. Like dualistic conceptions in general, this one is far too limiting.

The dualism written into state laws, and the structure of the medical profession, is also restrictive. Structural dualism, in this case, defines who is permitted to treat patients. Practicing medicine without a license, for example, is a crime. The purpose of such laws is ostensibly to protect the public. The result, however, is that the power, privilege, and resources of biomedicine are protected. In effect, these values block the legitimate use of other, non-specific, approaches to healing, especially by persons who are not certified as medical professionals. In this demonstration of dualism, there is also a sequence of either-or distinctions. The first asserts that there is scientific and non-scientific medicine; second, the former is legitimate and the latter non-legitimate; and third, scientific medicine is real and non-scientific treatment is fake. Any practice of medicine that is not scientific, therefore, cannot be efficacious, is potentially dangerous, and should be eliminated. Dualism is instrumental is generating absolutism, exclusiveness, and, where resources are involved, privilege.

There is also a humorous side to the circularity of the argument that dualism imposes on health, as found in a February 10, 1994, quote from the *New England Journal of Medicine*. "A resident's answer to the question: 'what is a well person?'—'A well person is a patient who has not been completely worked up'" [13, p. 440].

Such structural dualism is particularly unfortunate in the case of chronic disease. In short, the flexibility that is needed to treat chronic illnesses is stifled by biomedicine. An explicit division of labor, exclusivity of knowledge bases, the blatant disregard for subjectivity, and the peripherialization of patients are failings of the biomedical model. And any proposals to improve the current medical system, and make it more socially responsive, will have to take seriously these shortcomings. Otherwise, medicine will continue to be guided by a philosophy and structure that are rigid, contrived, and divorced from real social conditions.

A NEW MEDICAL WORLD-VIEW

What is being called for is a general reorientation of medicine. This new direction would include the following elements:

1. The absolutism and exclusiveness of the dualistic approach should be abandoned, along with the resulting materialism and narrow view of causality. Life should no longer be thought to consist primarily of physical elements that are mechanically united.
2. The body and the world would have an interpretive texture, or be implicated thoroughly in a humanly constructed milieu. What this means is that cultural, socioeconomic, political, and other contextual factors cannot be neatly severed from illness.
3. Factors relevant to health and illness should be **expanded** in order to understand how illness occurs. With the person no longer treated as a bundle of physiology, a number of psychological, emotional, and volitional factors become relevant in explaining the onset and cure of an illness.
4. A new range of interventions, which were possibly dismissed before as unscientific, must be envisioned. These are treatments that are not, by tradition, only bodily but take into consideration the whole person. These cures are not indicative of quackery, simply because they do not fall within the realm sanctioned traditionally by medical professionals.

For this expansion to take place, a change in the medical "world-view" is necessary. Medicine is philosophy and an entirely new theoretical basis is needed. Facing the problems posed by the increased prevalence of chronicity, a few practical reforms will be insufficient. Without a radically new paradigm, changes will be enacted within the same old intellectual and organizational framework. The impact of any new policy will thus be truncated.

Encouraged by this new philosophy will be the expansion of knowledge bases, practices, remedies, and modes of intervention. And as a result of this conceptual shift, divergent definitions, expectations, and views of physical reality will be more readily accepted than in the past. New experiences can thus be more easily introduced into the medical process, so that care can be made socially and culturally sensitive. In this particular example, the special problems of age-relevant cohorts can receive appropriate attention.

In general, medical practice must be democratized. Certainly this is a political process, but one defined in the broadest sense. What is involved, in addition to the exercise of political will, is symbolic politics. There is no doubt that the hegemony of biomedicine was instituted by a practical means. Nonetheless, this dominance has been legitimized through the use of unique symbolism.

Following the challenge to dualism, the traditional norms of medical practice can no longer be accorded the status of mandates. The biomedical model is illustrated to represent a symbolic reality, rather than a scientific fact. Therefore, the practice of medicine can be expanded simply through the adoption of alternative symbolism, or new ways of conceiving medical practice. In this way, persons are free to fashion an image of medicine that is minimally indebted to the biomedical model. Activists may be needed to carry out this change, but the guidance of a non-dualistic theory is also essential for this task. In this book, this emerging paradigm is referred to as postmodern.

Cassell reminds readers that "Doctors do not treat chronic illnesses. The chronically ill treat themselves with the help of their physicians; the physician is part of the treatment. Patients are in charge of themselves" [4, p. 125]. For this reason, democratization is crucial to addressing chronic illness. Barriers to the patient's self-treatment must be rolled back. The point is that patients must guide medicine, rather than vice-versa. They must have the right to define illness, appropriate intervention, and outcome. As Cassell continues, "The chronically ill person's personality, character, intelligence, store of knowledge, previous experience, goals, relationships to the body, relationships to society and to others, socioeconomic status, living circumstances, quality of medical care, and relationship with the doctor(s) all influence the nature, content and adequacy of treatment. Doctors who are oblivious to these factors or who believe that they [are] not really important, risk doing a bad job" [4, p. 125]. Medical experts, in sum, must no longer dominate the medical team, as a result of controlling the knowledge and resources that are available to the patient. Of course, this is the aim of democratization.

The allocation of resources is not an ethereal process, but one that is thoroughly social. Patients, as citizens, can vote with their feet. The playing field, however, must be leveled. One cannot choose if there are no alternatives; real voting cannot take place if reality is legitimately imploded by the medical model. Opening up the medical system, through true democratization, will go a long way to bringing treatment closer to citizens and improving care.

THE BASICS OF DEMOCRATIZATION

Various projects have been proposed in the name of democratization, but mostly to control costs. By encouraging community control, the health care system could be monitored closely and abuses could be reduced. Public regulation of the medical-industrial complex, in other words, would temper the drive for profit and centralization exhibited by service providers [15].

Professional standards review organizations, health systems agencies, community-based health programs and treatment facilities, and, most recently, a raft of state health plans have been proposed to give consumers a voice in determining the growth of services and facilities. The problem with these earlier attempts at democratization, even the now famous Oregon Plan, is that a few strategies associated with democracy were simply grafted onto the prevailing system. The philosophical side of democratization was never explored, and thus the epistemological, social, and cultural prerequisites of democracy were never given any attention. As a result, control of the health care system was not moved any closer to the citizenry.

The authors of this book walk an awkward line. On the one hand, we are calling for the thorough democratization of health care institutions, but on the other we do not supply a cookbook that shows how to achieve this end. Giving such details would defeat the purpose of democracy. Nonetheless, various considerations are discussed that are essential for establishing the framework necessary for widespread democratization. In fact, this kind of discussion has been missing from prior attempts to make the health care system more responsive to the public.

In a democracy, citizens should not be at the edge of the polity, although this has come to be the case. Democracy is thus quite radical, according to the etymological meaning of this term. The people, in other words, are at the "root" of a democratic society. They are given the latitude to impose on themselves rules, regulations, and obligations. Self-government, simply put, is the norm. The argument in this book is that medicine should not be exempt from this process. Despite charges to the opposite made by defenders of professional autonomy and hierarchy, along with those defending other vested interests, ordinary persons do have the right to participate fully in the operation of the health care system. And the skills and resources required for this undertaking will become available once democratization is under way.

Democracy does not occur in a vacuum. Certain conditions must be met before this style of government is possible. A culture of democracy, simply put, must be established. What this means is that persons must have the knowledge, practical wherewithal, and accessibility to the levers of decision-making necessary for them to have control over their health. Patients must be autonomous. Without this background, democracy is just another name for the protection of power and privilege. In the case of medicine, this means patients are permitted to express themselves, but not to alter the basic structure of how health care is provided [16, 17]. But having the ability to be self-directed, no matter what direction is taken, is fundamental to a real democracy.

Medicine has been exempted from the current trend toward democratization. The workplace and the classroom, for example, have been viewed as improved because of the introduction of democracy [10, p. 17]. Nonetheless, medicine has remained aloof from the *vox populi*. Moving medicine in the direction of democracy, however, should not be viewed as unthinkable, although many powerful groups may be threatened by this course of action. Yet like other institutions, the operation of the health care system will be enhanced by this change.

By empowering persons in this way, medicine will become more socially responsible. Monitoring can be increased, while services can be delivered in a socially sensitive manner. Waste will be reduced, along with other factors that result from this institution drifting away from public view. With ordinary persons at the heart of the health care system, services are likely to reflect social need. Citizens will have the latitude to correct situations in the environment that make them sick, in addition to determining a suitable level of treatment. Nonetheless, the point is not simply to control expenditures, and thus focus on instrumental or logistical concerns, but to alter the rationale that underpins medicine. As opposed to restrictive economic or professional imperatives, the "will of the people" will sustain service delivery.

THE THRUST OF THE BOOK

Basic to this book is the idea that good theory is essential to a successful plan. Before the crisis in American health care can be appreciated, a proper conceptual scheme is required to analyze its breakdown. Detailing the limited relevance of the biomedical model can open the door for further critique, in addition to expanding the range of alternatives. Nonetheless, an adequate remedy must also be guided by an appropriate philosophy. In this case, democracy must be thoroughly grounded theoretically, so that new options are not identified as idealistic, inferiorized, and dismissed out of hand.

The following tack is taken in this book to fostering the democratization of medicine. In Chapter 2 the philosophical antecedents of the biomedical model are outlined. Chapters 3 and 4 are devoted to specifying the theoretical and practice sides respectively of the rise of scientific medicine. And in Chapter 5, the inability of biomedicine, or scientific medicine, to treat chronic illness is discussed. The growth of the older population, particularly three decades hence and thereafter until the middle of the next century, is expected to impose a crushing strain on the biomedical model. At this juncture, the case is made for holistic interventions, given the severe limitations of biomedicine. The need for and feasibility of alternatives are argued to be viable. Throughout the second half of this book the stage is prepared for the arrival of democratic medicine. A non-dualistic philosophical base of intervention is unveiled in Chapter 6. Subsequent to this démarche, the broad policy implications of anti-dualism that are illustrated in Chapter 7 can be appreciated. And finally, some key issues in the democratization of medical practice are assessed in the last chapter.

Clearly this book is informed by sociology and gerontology. On the other hand, however, at the core of this work is philosophy. These disciplines are not necessarily at odds, contrary to some mainstream thinking. Science, no matter what type, divorced from philosophy, has no substance or direction. But philosophy that is not anchored in concrete issues is pure speculation. Accordingly, the authors want to avoid both crude empiricism and ethereal philosophizing. Their goal has been to combine sociology, gerontology, and philosophy, so that a well conceived critique of the current crisis in medicine can be proffered [18]. Most important, this mode of criticism is not constrained by systemic imperatives that go unscrutinized. Hopefully, this end has been achieved and new insights have been gained into the application of medicine.

REFERENCES

1. E. G. Mishler, Viewpoint: Critical Perspectives on the Biomedical Model, in *Social Contexts of Health, Illness and Patient Care,* E. G. Mishler, L. R. Amarasingham, S. D. Osherson, S. T. Hauser, N. E. Waxler, and R. Liem (eds.), Cambridge University Press, Cambridge, pp. 1-23, 1981.
2. D. M. Fox, *Power and Illness: The Failure and Future of American Health Policy,* University of California Press, Berkeley, 1993.
3. L. Foss and K. Rothenberg, *The Second Medical Revolution,* Shambhala, Boston, pp. 42-71, 1987.
4. E. J. Cassell, *The Nature of Suffering and the Goals of Medicine,* Oxford University Press, New York, 1991.
5. K. Pellitier, *Holistic Medicine,* Delacorte Press, San Francisco, 1979.
6. J. H. Knowles, Introduction to "Doing Better and Feeling Worse: Health in the United States," *Daedalus, 106,* pp. v-vi, 1977.
7. S. R. Graubard, Preface to "Doing Better and Feeling Worse: Health in the United States," *Daedalus, 106,* pp. 1-9, 1977.
8. A. Waldovski, Doing Better and Feeling Worse: The Political Pathology of Health Policy, *Daedalus, 106,* 1977.
9. E. D. Pellegrino and D. C. Thomasma, *The Virtues in Medical Practice,* Oxford University Press, New York, 1993.
10. D. Reisman, *Market and Health,* St. Martin's Press, New York, 1993.

11. J. M. Morse and J. L. Johnson, Understanding the Illness Experience, in *The Illness Experience,* M. Morse and J. L. Johnson (eds.), Sage Publications, Newbury Park, California, pp. 1-12, 1991.
12. B. J. Good, *Medicine, Rationality and Experience,* Cambridge University Press, Cambridge, pp. 127ff, 1994.
13. C. K. Meador, Occasional Notes: The Last Well Person, *New England Journal of Medicine,* February 10, 1994.
14. E. G. Mishler, Social Contexts, of Health Care, in *Social Contexts of Health, Illness, and Patient Care,* E. G. Mishler, L. R. Amarasingham, S. D. Osherson, S. T. Hauser, N. E. Waxler, and R. Liem (eds.), Cambridge University Press, Cambridge, pp. 141-168, 1981.
15. J. Braverman, *Crisis in Health Care,* Acropolis Books, Washington, D.C., pp. 119-145, 1978.
16. J. Vanek (ed.), *Self-management,* Penguin Books, Middlesex, England, 1975.
17. H. C. Boyte, H. Booth, and S. Max, *Citizen Action and the New American Populism,* Temple University Press, Philadelphia, 1986.
18. H. Marcuse, *One-dimensional Man,* Beacon Press, Boston, p. 148, 1964.

The Shift from Speculation to Science

RELIGION AND SCIENCE

The aim of this chapter is to illustrate that the biomedical model does not exist in a vacuum. Furthermore, medicalization does not consist simply of the application of increasingly sophisticated procedures and techniques. What each of these approaches presupposes is an image of the individual, valid knowledge, the focus of intervention, causality, and so forth, which underpin modern medical treatment. Understanding the current predicament in health care, accordingly, requires that insight be gained into this tacit side of medicine. This might be referred to as the silent or hidden dimension of the biomedical model.

The underside of modern medicine has been referred to by Foucault as the "man-the-Machine" model [1, p. 136]. As described by Leder, the "medical body comes to be viewed not primarily as purpose and ensouled; nor as the scene of moral dramas; nor as a place wherein cosmological and social forces gather; but simply as an intricate machine" [2, p. 3]. Therefore, approaching the person as a composite of physical forces makes sense; using science and technology to fix the body is only logical.

But this mechanical analogy, however, is a relatively recent development. Persons were not always stripped of mystery. Spirits and demons were once a vital part of human existence; life was replete with uncertainty. Taming the body, along with other aspects of life, however, came to be viewed as a sign of progress and welcomed. The discipline enforced by science, as Foucault writes, joined the "analyzable body to the manipulable body" [1, p. 136]. A person is thus available who can be rendered docile and inspected.

Yet, from the early Greeks to the end of the medieval period, medical intervention was quite convoluted. Any complaint could be the result of a combination of factors, both natural and spiritual. As King notes, gods controlled nature, thus creating a difficult situation for the physician [3]. In short, where does the cause of events reside? With regard to medicine, should a physical ailment be blamed on god or nature? Clearly, operating within such an environment was quite difficult. Precision was a very elusive quality.

Should a physician try to appease the gods or address issues related to human physiology? In point of fact, many of the remedies that were proposed were designed to deal with both concerns. For central to any cure is "the personal relationship between god and the particular patient" [3, p. 13]. Gods do not bring about a cure, but they determine which remedies are effective. Knowing a god's involvement in nature was thus essential to promoting health or eradicating illness.

Early on, medicine was thought to be a part of a unique cosmos. The will of gods infiltrated every aspect of life. Mystical forces, hidden causes, and cryptic signs were operative everywhere. A physician, therefore, had to be both a soothsayer and technician. Both meditation and technical skill were necessary to produce a cure. At this juncture, the practice of medicine was sustained by a defending God's goodness and omnipotence in view of the existence of evil.

But gradually the move was away from metaphysics and toward science. Myth and speculation were supposed to be replaced by fact. Direct observation, logical analysis, and the dissection of nature were to be elevated in importance. The reason for this shift of attention was quite simple: scientific medicine would be much more effective. As a result of concentrating only on factors that could be directly observed, treatment would improve. By eliminating the unknown, a source of serious error would be eliminated. A right and wrong way could then be clearly established for identifying and remedying a problem. King characterizes this as the move from religion to scientific medicine [3].

Yet, this change did not occur all at once. Although the influence of gods gradually diminished with the passage of time, pure nature was not understood to exist for quite awhile. Hippocrates might have been an advocate of science, but the conditions necessary to envision natural laws would not be available until *circa* 1600. To varying degrees, the admixture of nature and spirit continued throughout western history until the arrival of Descartes. The metaphysical and physical were intermingled until he made his famous theoretical stratagem. And some writers, such as Richard Zaner, claim that Descartes' shift toward mind/body dualism was not complete, [4] which is a point taken up in Chapter 3.

What is vital to appreciate is that a science of medicine would not be possible, as long as nature remained contaminated by wild speculation about the presence of gods or spirits. To use Carolyn Merchant's phrase, the "death of nature" was required for the success of science [5]. Regularities, patterns, and laws would be obscured, or misinterpreted, by a concern for salvation, fate, or destiny. In order for science to develop, unencumbered access to nature must be possible. The purpose in nature must be able to be directly apprehended, without the distortion that results from extraneous considerations. Richard Zaner describes this process when he states that the purpose of medicine is to explain maladies "without reference to persons, souls, psyches, spirits, minds, or even social life" [6].

Up until the arrival of Descartes, material doctrines were joined with claims about spirits that acted on organs. Metaphors were used that suggested the body is animated by little known forces. Galen, for instance, talked about various *pneuma* that drove the circulation of blood. Assorted "faculty" promoted growth and decay. On the other hand, Paracelsus looked to the stars to explain water-balance [3, p. 116]. And alchemists, as is well known, thought that magic played a large role in altering the basic elements, so as to form new ones. In each example, nature is adulterated.

Critics argued that knowledge would not progress until nature is deanimated, or transformed into a "plenum of passive matter driven by mechanical forces" [7, p. 20]. Chaos would reign until nature is treated as an inert object. Following the objectification of nature, a true science of medicine could be engendered. Laws of intervention could be discovered pertaining to every facet of care. Hylozoism, the early Greek belief that all matter has life, and other teleologies could thus be replaced by more sound principles of development. The dark recesses concealed by metaphysics would finally be open for direct examination; the light of day would be able to penetrate to the core of life. Facts combined with judicious reasoning would be the cornerstone of medicine. Accordingly, medicine would finally achieve a new level of respectability. Instead of propitiating "natural powers," physicians would concentrate on restoring the natural harmony of organisms.

THE MATERIALIZATION OF EXISTENCE

Key to sound clinical judgments are unbiased observation, accurate measurement, and a straightforward plan of action. This kind of precision is not possible when the clinical setting is sullied by vital spirits and other vaguely known powers. The "medical gaze," as Foucault writes, must not be clouded by faith or myth [8, p. 16]. For a true scientist is guided by nothing other than the facts of a case. In terms of medicine, this conclusion has come to mean that reliable knowledge has an organic source.

The focus of attention, therefore, was directed to the "epistemological primacy of the corpse" [7, p. 22]. The person is thus envisioned to be a piece of meat; the physician is an explorer who traverses a novel physiological realm. Suffering is speculative, while pain is equated with the present physical state of the body. Eric Cassell makes this point when he remarks that a corpse has no purpose, as exemplified by "desires, affections, wishes and choices" [9, p. 244]. As he goes on to say, "disease, then, is something an organ has; illness is something a man has" [10, p. 48].

Consistent with the prevailing trend, physicians in the seventeenth century became more realistic [11]. A concerted effort was made to restrict input to physical observations. Only factors that could be directly apprehended would be introduced as evidence. In this way, the influence of metaphysics would be curtailed. Only so-called hard data would be involved in making a clinical decision. In general, physicians became empiricists.

As opposed to assumptions, opinions, and beliefs, empiricists base knowledge on experience. Through strict observation and experimentation, data are recorded. No commentary is supposed to be offered. Indeed, perception is never to stray from the physical evidence [12, p. 33]. In this sense, the mind is trained to operate like a blank slate, thereby copying *verbatim* the physical reality of events. "Objective observers," notes Engel, "regard nature as independent from themselves and unaffected by their act of observation" [13, p. 117].

With regard to the practice of medicine, the acceptance of empiricism required that the former image of the body be transformed. Humors, lacuna, and other dark spaces would have to be purged from descriptions of human anatomy. The body, simply put, would have to be rendered transparent. Imagination must not be allowed to interfere with obtaining a clear picture of the body. Therefore, human existence had to be systematically demythologized.

What this meant was that the body was transformed into a thing. Given the adoption of empiricism, making this change was not difficult. If only objective or concrete information was to be treated as valid, the body could not be exempted from this rule. Human physiology, accordingly, had to be stripped of all non-empirical elements. As a result, the body was thoroughly materialized. The Germans have a word to depict the resulting body—*Körper*. This version of the *soma* consists of inert, dead matter. A person's existence is thus nothing more than an organic mass. At the basis of life are chemical compounds, biochemical reactions, and various structural components. Anything else is considered to be conjecture.

The complete materialization of life was made possible by a theoretical maneuver inaugurated by Descartes but expanded upon and fulfilled by his followers. In his search for certainty in knowledge, he created a dualistic system that is still at the core of modern medicine. According to Jonas, Cartesianism is the philosophy that "carried the mind of man from the vitalistic monism of early times to the materialistic monism" of today [14, p. 12]. Descartes set out to establish an Archimedean point, devoid of the usual metaphysical overtones. Not only was a firm base of knowledge proposed, but the justification became available for approaching the body as something that is simply corporeal. Following Descartes, the body should not be viewed as sacred or mysterious.

The thrust of Descartes' position is that the mind (*res cogitans*) could be severed from the body (*res extensa*) [15, pp. 201-202]. His point is that everything non-material should be understood as removed categorically from the material realm. Matter is thus freed from contaminants; pristine matter is thus available for inspection. Due to this separation, those who are pursuing truth cannot be tricked by uncertainties. The body is now completely accessible to the senses. For this reason, Descartes is known as the harbinger of light [8, p. xiii]. Mind, spirit, consciousness, or soul, for example, cannot compromise the search for knowledge. In effect, the influence of these intangible elements is neutralized.

Hence the body gains a sense of autonomy. Like nature, the body becomes an object that is encountered. Actually, the body comes to be viewed as simply another part of nature, which could be prodded, probed, or rearranged in any number of ways. Most importantly is that the prospect finally existed for discovering laws related to biochemistry and other aspects of physiology. With the body materialized, medicine could at last become a *bona fide* science.

No one should be surprised, therefore, that the body came to be viewed as a machine. To be sure, this is a favorite metaphor of physicians. Descartes believed this imagery was appropriate, along with Thomas Boyle, Friedrich Hoffman, and La Mettrie [4, p. 119]. About the same time, Harvey applied this outlook to conceptualizing the circulation of blood. Later on, life was thought to be predicated on a series of molecular "building blocks." As part of this trend, and extending the logic of homeostasis, metabolism became the focus of attention. And finally, the study of so-called "giant molecules"—proteins, nucleic acids, and enzymes—and genetic mechanisms were thought to have promise for unveiling the source of life [16].

In each stage, the body is assumed to be a complete and self-contained system. The directions, control mechanisms, and means for growth have a material rationale. As an interlocking network of causes and functions, the body is readily available for observation and intervention. Nature may be complex, but with enough effort its laws can be exposed. While the body may be opaque, there is nothing fundamentally occult about its operation. The body is an example of "indifferent extension" or, stated differently, a material field that is immediately accessible for the universal application of medical techniques [14, pp. 18, 35]. As a lifeless mechanism, examination, classification, and intervention should proceed with little difficulty.

Rather than the cosmos, modern medicine is based on a "culture of science" [17]. This phrase suggests that science is not value-free, as its advocates claim, but is sustained by a particular set of values. At the core of this culture is the dualism that was outlined by Descartes. That the body can be controlled, similar to nature, is a direct product of the bifurcation believed to exist between mind and body. To use Heidegger's language, the body is a "standing reserve"—a mass and resource—that can be regulated according to laws of nature [18, p. 19].

Once inside this culture, many of the beliefs and practices adhered to by physicians make sense. What might appear to be unethical or dehumanizing behavior, within the confines of the culture of science is not only deemed acceptable but also is encouraged. For example, mechanical, chemical, and other abstract imagery is identified as progressive. Cause and effect puzzles challenge physicians, yet like nature their secrets will eventually be known. But in the end, patients do not even resemble the humans who are otherwise relatives, friends, and neighbors. Roland Barthes' observation is noteworthy at this juncture: the transparencies found in physiology textbooks are clear and informative but strip the body of human significance and dignity [19].

Every dimension is exposed for dissection; every layer of human existence is peeled away nicely.

FACT AND TRUTH

Physicians are expected to make correct decisions about ailments. Facts must be gathered and diagnoses verified. Presupposed by biomedicine is a correct mode of intervention. At the root of every problem are physiological processes that can be apprehended, if observation and reason are unobstructed. This concern for perceptual acuity, accordingly, places medicine at the center of an epistemological controversy.

Of primary concern is the status of facts and reality. In other words, are facts interpretive or are they things? Is the identity of facts strictly empirical, or are culture, context, biography, and other idiosyncrasies relevant to gathering valid knowledge? In the example of medicine, the issue is whether primacy should be given to physiological markers when attempting to make a diagnosis. Clearly, vital to achieving accuracy in any endeavor is the ability to differentiate fact from illusion. But isolating and pinpointing the cause of a disease especially requires close attention to detail, for a life may hang in the balance. Indeed, precision is a quality that is cherished by practically every physician.

A lot of time and money are spent trying to record bodily signs in order to reach a high standard of diagnostic reliability [20, p. 38]. Of course, this strategy should be expected, given the assumption of mind-body dualism. For attendant to this differentiation is the separation of objectivity from subjectivity, or, in more modern parlance, fact from value. As might be expected, objectivity is associated with extension, while subjectivity pervades cognition. Because of this distinction facts are "externalized," similar to the body [21, p. 4]. Traditionally, this maneuver has been considered beneficial, for diagnostic input can be judged dispassionately.

Although Cartesianism is thought to reflect reality, this is not exactly the case. Instead, various assumptions are introduced that support a particular version of knowledge. In short, asymmetry is tacitly accepted as existing between objectivity and subjectivity. And due to this skewed relationship, cognition is systematically inferiorized; "everyday experience is ignored and denigrated as illusory, subjective, and shallow" [22, p. 137].

As a result of his anxiety about being tricked by an "evil genius," Descartes argued that the origin of knowledge should be removed from human control [23]. True knowledge is timeless and thus enduring, while opinion is evanescent. Hence, persons should strive to purge themselves of all opinions, in order to enhance perception. On the surface this may appear to be sound advice. Problems begin to arise, however, when subjectivity is equated with opinion. To be specific, the human element must be sacrificed in the pursuit of knowledge.

Descartes claims that in order to perceive things "clearly and distinctly," detachment is necessary. Passion and similar emotions must be moved to the periphery of the knowledge acquisition process. Subjectivity thus becomes a liability—an impulsive factor that can wreak havoc at any moment. Without any warning or reason, subjectivity can appear and distort perception. Other insubstantial considerations may sabotage the collection of true knowledge, but for Descartes subjectivity is clearly a major source of confusion and thus evil. Anything related to "inwardness," therefore, should be eschewed. In this regard, Bordo writes that "Cartesianism is nothing if not a passion for separation, purification, and demarcation" [23, p. 17]. Only by interrogating the *res extensa,* categorically removed from the influence of the mind, can accurate knowledge be obtained.

In actual practice, this conclusion means that facts must not be viewed to have any connection with subjectivity. Science is grounded on the "basic rule of the empiricist schools that all knowledge has to prove itself through the *sense certainty* of systematic observation that secures intersubjectivity" [24, p. 74]. Accordingly, facts have been described as sense impressions, stimuli, and other discrete pieces of bits of data. Consistent with Descartes admonition, facts have been "denatured," or removed from any human context that would restrict their applicability [8, p. 16]. True facts have been portrayed as not having any human characteristics. In this way, becoming objective would not be impossible, because factors uncontaminated by cognition do exist. If an individual were properly trained, a purely empirical datum could be garnered.

Empirical indicators were gradually equated with objectivity. Furthermore, as Rorty correctly notes, objective knowledge came to be treated as a by-product of accurately "mirroring" nature [25]. Like a camera, a trained mind could mimic the empirical surface of reality. Harking back to Locke, empirical traits are imagined to be imprinted on the mind. Empirical facts are material and autonomous. As a consequence of this dualism, the senses are overwhelmed by reality. Clearly, epistemological security is guaranteed by establishing facts on an empirical bedrock.

At the same time, subjectivity is discredited as a place to find true knowledge. All that emanates from there, instead, is interpretation that obscures objectivity. Subjectivity is the source of error that must be overcome, if reliable knowledge is ever to be uncovered. Anything that is tainted by subjectivity, such as values, beliefs, or commitments, must be expelled from research. Because interpretation is very volatile, subjective knowledge claims are uncertain. And such unpredictability is not supposed to be a part of science.

Assumed by this rendition of facts is the correspondence theory of truth. According to this thesis, truth is defined as *adaequatio rei et intellectus*. Simply put, this phrase is usually translated to mean that the mind approximates reality. An objective referent, in other words, is necessary to verify any claim; subjectivity is not capable of self-validation. Anything a person might say, for example, is meaningless unless it can be corroborated by empirical evidence. As with facts, the criteria for truth are exteriorized. Hence persons are deprived of the ability to investigate or question the basis of truth. Rather, they have only the latitude to recognize their errors and make the required correctives. Adjustment to reality is expected.

As should be noted, becoming objective requires that all personal interests be renounced [26, p. 119]. Subsequent to the acceptance of dualism, the pursuit of truth demands that even the self be abandoned. Opinions, emotions, and personal insights have no validity, until they can be tied to empirical data. And if this validation is not immediately forthcoming, these phenomena must be dismissed as fictitious.

In this Cartesian search for concreteness, facts and truth are severed from human contact. These factors are utilized, in turn, to judge behavior. Moreover, throughout this process the impact of interpretation is ignored. Knowledge is thus purified and transformed into something constant, universal, and worthy of veneration. Facts do not reflect conviction, but a perspicuous (external) reality. Personal defects are not allowed to defile the encounter with facts. Human weakness cannot jeopardize the quest for truth. Without a doubt, this was Descartes' aim and a goal shared currently by most modern physicians.

Within this context, reliance on an ever increasing armamentarium of high-tech diagnostic and therapeutic devices is understandable [2, p. 2]. In the mid-1800s, the promise of objectivity became real because of the development of new diagnostic instruments, such as the stethoscope, ophthalmoscope, and laryngoscope. And the microscope and x-ray, for example, certainly enhanced the prospects for dispassionate examination [27, pp. 136-137]. Physicians no longer have to touch the body, but merely monitor certain dials and screens. As Descartes would desire, reason would thus not be defiled by contact with the flesh.

Particularly following the widespread onset of computerization, these technical approaches are thought to garner objective data. Computers, after all, are presumed to be unemotional and able to organize information without bias; computers epitomize the exercise of reason. Human sources of error are believed to be controlled, because the clinical setting is systematically regulated. Therefore, physicians can have, at their disposal, facts as opposed to simply feelings and other flimsy kinds of input.

CAUSES AND ACTIONS

The impetus to action has always been a mystery. In other words, what is the rationale for an object's movement? Why should movement begin or continue along a particular path? Typically, answers to these questions have made reference to a "vital spirit," "first cause," "demiurge," "*telos,*" or some other metaphysical force. An ethereal element is cited in each case as responsible for inaugurating a series of events. Metaphysics is intimately tied to matter. The problem with these responses is that no insight is gained into the origin of motion. An abstraction is simply invoked to address a very complex issue, and ambiguity is allowed to plague causality.

As might be expected, movement was reconceptualized following the acceptance of dualism. Unverifiable sources of action had to be abandoned. Similar to the body, facts and truth, the justification for movement was also materialized. Specifically, the idea of mechanical causality gained widespread acceptance.

To borrow from Weber, action was "rationalized" [28, pp. 84-85]. Through the application of quantitative measures, the guesswork was removed from comprehending movement. The position of force, along with an explanation for direction, velocity and momentum, was provided with exact parameters. Descriptions became very concrete, as discussions revolved around "causal chains" and "webs of causation" [29]. As opposed to a *telos,* for example, a mechanical cause has a precise location, impact, and *raison d'être.* Accordingly, adopting causal imagery would foster progress in science, for the universe could be assumed to have a structural design. Husserl describes the thrust of true causality as follows: "All that is together in the world has a universal immediate or mediate way of belonging together" [30, p. 31]. In other words, cosmic or spiritual forces are replaced by more substantial reasons for order. Placing an emphasis on structure tends to deanimate the identity and relationship between events. After all, structures are inert.

Many advantages are attendant to causal explanations. For example, essentialism can be abandoned. Prior to the use of causal imagery, there was much speculation about the preternatural kernel of objects. Did matter have a destiny, vital core, or some organizational secret that must be unveiled? When searching for a cause, however, these speculative concerns become inconsequential. Most important about a cause are its physical characteristics, such as mass. For within a causal framework action results from a collision between forces. Hence elements that are immaterial have no relevance, because their impact cannot be measured. Therefore, viewed as a cause an object has no traits other than those that can be assigned a mathematical value and spatial location. An object's identity is thus solidified.

Additionally, the relationship that exists between entities is no longer vague. A divine plan, for example, is outmoded as an explanation. Instead, material contact, usually thought to consist of attraction and repulsion, holds events and objects together. The strength of this association, moreover, is calculated in terms of force vectors that are concrete and readily accessible. In this sense, reality is united by material ties. The so-called "power of explanation" can be determined through rigorous research and outlined in terms of laws of probability. Given the position of A, a certain likelihood can be specified that B will be affected in a particular way.

Due to the concrete quality of causality, a neat ordering of events is also possible. Without referring to time, mind, or reason, for example, objects can be arranged *ad seriatim* and dealt with individually [31]. Again, because of the emphasis placed on materialism, the logic of causality is not arcane. Subsequent to examining nature closely, the proper organization of causal linkages becomes obvious. A cause, in other words, can be distinguished easily from an effect, so that gradually a series of correctly positioned "If . . . then" statements can be proposed.

Nothing is left to conjecture. The cosmos is transformed into a causal mechanism, with all of its components integrated into a unified whole. A key achievement for scientists is that now a well-defined locus of intervention can be pinpointed. With a causal chain completely circumscribed, the purpose of each link can be known. Accurate predictions are thus made possible, because the element of chance is eliminated from each equation. Rather than spontaneous or random, action is understood to reside within an orderly system of influences.

Remember, the thrust of science is often claimed to be prediction and control. And conceptualizing the relationship between particles, atoms, or larger things as causal is assumed to foster this end. Because causes and their effects are inextricably joined by material connectors, the chances of developing a unified theory of nature are presumed to greatly improve.

The search for "magic bullets," for example, to cure disease is thoroughly justified. With causes readily identifiable, a researcher can zero in on the single factor that produces a malady. And subsequent to the acceptance of germ theory and the development of vaccines for a host of afflictions, this end seemed realizable. In this regard, Paul Starr argues that the focus on bacteriology is a prime example of looking for an isolated cause of disease [27, p. 189]. Streamlined models were thus developed and became commonplace, which overlooked the competing claims that relate to the social side of illness.

Physicians have had a penchant for the "specific etiology" thesis, which is dependent on the ability to isolate specific causes of events. And furthermore, as Dubos writes, "biochemical lesions, molecular pathology, congenital anomalies, and genetic disorders are direct linear descendants of the doctrine of specificity" [32, p. 326]. Each of these factors is physical and, with the proper tools and preparation, readily visible. According to this causal outlook, both external and internal agents are thought to impinge on a properly functioning body, thereby disrupting proper functioning. Doctors support this way of thinking, claims Engel, because these causes can be easily attacked and destroyed [33].

NORMS AND EQUILIBRIUM

A perennial question pertains to the content of norms. Stated simply, what range of events should be expected? In more social terms, what moral behavior is normative? At issue is the baseline that should be used to judge whether an event or action is acceptable.

The Western tradition is replete with abstractions employed to convey a sense of normativeness. The mean, justice (*Dike*) and the "middle way" are classic examples of this approach to clarifying norms. But of course, these ideas are unverifiable, and thus normative standards remain uncertain and debatable. Therefore, nothing but faith is available to forestall the sudden proliferation of norms and the accompanying chaos.

As part of the general move toward the materialization of every facet of life, particularly subsequent to the onset of evolutionary theory, norms have been described with respect to equilibrium. Essential to the principle of equilibrium is a natural center, around which an organism or nature equilibrates. Survival, in fact, depends on maintaining a fine balance between the parts of the natural or social body. At an optional level of functioning, a "balance of forces" is present [34, p. 17].

Without this center, evolution could fly off in any direction. There would be no governor to prevent development from following a tangent that would end in entropy. A path might be taken, in short, that terminates in complete exhaustion and collapse. Diverging too far from the norm, or core of sustenance, would be devastating.

The point is that change is natural, and thus inherent correctives exist to insure that growth is not disruptive. Uniformity is generated by an internal mechanism that guarantees the proper rate and direction of development. A moving equilibrium is protected, with deviations kept within a fairly narrow range. Any movement that strays too far from the center is checked and redirected back toward the norm.

Particularly noteworthy is that the notion of immanence is demythologized in the equilibrium model [35, p. 157]. As opposed to searching for some primordial guidepost, or "evolving potential," balance is assessed by observing the units of the system. By looking at the *relationship* between these components any irregularity can be detected. Strains or conflicts can be witnessed directly at the nexus of elements. There is no need to hypothesize about the stability of a cosmic pattern, for example. Assessing equilibrium, instead, is understood to be purely an empirical issue.

Hence, a normative state is not rarefied. Variability is measured and regulated with regard to the confluence of elements within a system. Change is intra-systemic. Stability is not a mythical problem but is related to bringing various structures into harmony. Rather than concealed, norms reside at the intersection of these obtrusive factors. Accordingly, clear context is provided to evaluate any phase of movement. Norms are thus tangible and easily recognized. Both nature and society are thought to be gravitating toward a denouement that can be readily monitored.

As a consequence of concretizing norms, the causes of change can be isolated and plotted. When norms are abstract, deviation is difficult, if not impossible, to detect. Deprived of a testable baseline, how can the direction of change be known with any certainty? Motion may be witnessed, but little can be said about its status. Is a specific state favorable or detrimental? Answering this question presupposes a particular point of reference that can be examined. An equilibrium path can then be charted, so that evaluations can be made about the need for any corrections. The comparisons can be made that are necessary to recognize progression of digressions [36]. Determining the health or illness of such a system, accordingly, is not a metaphysical undertaking.

From a scientific point of view, an important consequence is that a departure from the norm can be detected the moment it occurs. Considering this possibility, discovering the etiology of a deviation is within reach. Once a boundary is delimited, the course of a breach can be exposed. The rationale for this disturbance may not be readily visible, but through experimentation relevant information can be obtained. As opposed to something spiritual, a material cause can be studied.

In the late nineteenth and early twentieth century, this focus on equilibrium culminated research on DNA, RNA, and proteins related to cell growth and replication [20, p. 170]. These phenomena are understood to be the "keys" to the evolutionary process, and hold the secrets to preventing various physical illness and social problems. "The essence of aliveness," write Foss and Rothenberg, "was thought to be reducible to [these] organismic fundamentals" [20, p. 170]. Consistent with both evolutionary theory and the equilibrium model, organic growth is assumed to fluctuate around these core elements. Gaining insight into the DNA molecule, accordingly, would be sufficient to make a quantum leap in medicine. Nothing, in short, would be beyond the grasp of medical science, once genetic engineering is perfected.

TECHNĒ OR PERCEPTION?

Becoming anti-metaphysical was thought to usher in a new era in understanding norms. Bias and dogma would be rejected in favor of fact. Speculation would be ended, with attention directed to reality. The overall quality of life would thereby be improved, because a reliable stock of knowledge would be available to development. Nature, the interface between persons and the environment, and interpersonal relationships could be enhanced. Natural laws and moral codes could be unearthed and reinforced.

Clearly, basing social life on reason, rather than faith, myth, prejudice, or tyrannical authority, would be beneficial. This project of the Enlightenment made perfect sense, until the human was identified as problematic. When the person became a source of prejudice and error, the promise of science began to be questioned. Apparently, becoming scientific requires the liquidation of the human quotient. If subjectivity is also indicative of metaphysics, interpretation is a threat to progress. As part of degrading subjectivity, the human element would have to be removed from every endeavor, if high levels of efficiency and effectiveness were ever to be attained.

According to the basic tenets of Cartesian dualism, subjectivity is as worthless as the soul, God, or Divine Right. Cognitive activity, therefore, cannot be a valid source of knowledge. Inwardness, explains Tillich, undermines logic, reason, and sound judgement [37, p. 76]. In the pursuit of knowledge, cognition became recognized as anathema to truth. The thinking and intuitive subject, engaged in various quotidian affairs, is capricious and had to be controlled.

Nonetheless, dualists persist in the belief that subjectivity is a contaminant and should be avoided, and try continually to overcome the influence of personal bias. But how is knowledge supposed to be collected? How can scientists proceed if their mere presence jeopardizes the scientific endeavor? If scientists cannot be objective, their contribution to the accumulation of knowledge is appreciably reduced. They will have to take a place along side those they criticize, such as priests, shamans, and other visionaries. This demotion, however, would be devastating to the stature of science. Science would not deserve the privileged position usually reserved for it in the hierarchy of academic disciplines.

This quandary has been resolved by an appeal to methodology. In other words, through the use of a particular style of methodology, human influence in research is imagined to be minimized. Because quantitative methods are assumed to be devoid of values, they are touted to deanimate the research setting. Jacques Ellul contends that the strength of this sort of technology, or *technē,* is its ability to perpetrate the illusion of neutrality. His point is that "technique alone is rigorously objective. It blots out all personal opinions" [38, p. 131].

To a certain extent, research is guided by scientific methodology. Biases and presuppositions are peripherialized, because quantitative methods are operationalized as a series of step-wise instructions. And because these guidelines are neat and concise, and do not necessarily involve interpretation, subjectivity appears to be exorcised. By focusing on what are considered to be self-evident techniques, the human element is obscured.

Technē has reached levels never before imagined. The production of increasingly advanced software and hardware, such as expert systems, has illustrated to the public the limited relevance of the human element [39]. In short, practically any task can be improved through the introduction of high-tech instruments designed to perform tasks formerly undertaken by humans. A computer, for example, is not emotional, does not have a bad day, and thus is unquestionably reliable.

At the root of this headlong rush to adopt technology is the issue of "trained perception." Simply put, humans are believed to be unpredictable, due to faulty reasoning and fluctuating perceptual acuity. Therefore, they should not be trusted to make crucial decisions. Their capabilities can be improved, however, by having data identified, sorted, and analyzed by various technical means. Through the use of these devices, humans receive the support required for them to overcome their weaknesses.

With the assistance of quantitative procedures, the effects of subjectivity are thought to be curtailed. An analytic strategy is instituted that ostensibly does not involve interpretation. Real objectivity is at hand, once a few techniques are mastered. Technical precision is substituted for perception; cognition is replaced by calculation. Gradually the human mind is equated with methodological practices that search for information in a manner unaffected by personal foibles and situational contingencies [40].

It should be noted that this faith in *technē* is underpinned by dualism. By becoming more and more formalized, methodological techniques are treated as if they are divorced from interpretation. Not only is this schism possible, but it is encouraged. In fact, the future of science appears to be tied to technological innovation. Once methodology is thoroughly mechanized, error will be a thing of the past. The exercise of reason will no longer be stifled by poor quality data.

THE WORLD-VIEW OF SCIENTIFIC MEDICINE

As will be discussed in the next chapter, the biomedical model is the centerpiece of the current practice of medicine. But viewing humans as physio-chemical organisms is not necessarily natural. Instead, several preconditions must be met before this image makes sense. Dualism, for example, must be firmly entrenched, before treating the body as an object is justified. The philosophical considerations raised in this chapter provide the essential background, or *"epistēmē"* as Foucault might say, for biological medicine. This epistemological grid constitutes the philosophy that "make[s] possible the appearance of objects during a given period of time" [41, p. 33], which in this case is the modern medical tradition. Without this philosophical backdrop, in other words, biomedicine would be difficult, if not impossible, to justify.

Stated another way, modern medicine has been established through a subtle form of "cultural authority." According to Starr, "cultural authority entails the construction of reality through definitions of fact and value" [27, p. 13]. The definitions that have been adopted in this case can be traced back to Descartes, with various modifications and improvements along the way. In the end, medicine has become wrapped in a conceptual scheme that provides it with credibility and enormous power.

This is not to argue that these considerations brought biomedicine into existence. While recalling Weber's discussion of the relationship between Protestantism and Capitalism, a causal link cannot be said to be present between dualism or the equilibrium thesis and the biomedical model [42]. Nonetheless, these and other tenets supported the advent of biomedicine. Without a particular constellation of underlying ideas, the prevailing rendition of medicine would not likely have come to fruition.

Germane at this juncture is that modern medicine rests on a unique vision. But this viewpoint is not innocent. Critics contend that biomedicine is dehumanizing, for humans are treated as homunculi. Biological reductionism occurs that results in associating medical problems with material or physical causes. Remedies, moreover, are mostly proposed that affect these physical sources of disease. As a result, the range of interventions is fairly narrow.

In general, life is materialized. Ideals, notes Lyotard, are supplanted by a focus on skills [43, p. 48]. Therefore, questions that have to do with value or purpose are considered to be irrelevant, given this limited orientation, and any talk about change will likely be restricted to technical matters. Any attempt to reorient medicine will be considered extravagant and unworkable; something that involves values that cannot be reconciled.

Reversing this trend is not merely a matter of deploying medical technology or fiscal resources in novel ways. Much more important may be rethinking the general philosophy that supports biomedicine.

Edmund Husserl offered this strategy as a solution to the dehumanizing effects of science he was witnessing in Europe during the 1930s [44]. Although his proposal is insightful, the focus has remained on pragmatic fixes. Yet without exploring the impact of the assumptions of biomedicine, rearranging current medical practices will probably be of minor importance. Regardless of this criticism, those who want to comprehend thoroughly the biomedical model should delve deeper than its surface characteristics.

REFERENCES

1. M. Foucault, *Discipline and Punish: The Birth of the Prison,* Vintage, New York, 1979.
2. D. Leder, Introduction, in *The Body in Medical Thought and Practice,* D. Leder (ed.), Kluwer, Dordrecht, 1992.
3. L. S. King, *The Growth of Medical Thought,* University of Chicago Press, Chicago, 1963.
4. R. M. Zaner, *Ethics and the Clinician Encounter,* Prentice-Hall, Englewood Cliffs, New Jersey, 1988.
5. C. Merchant, *The Death of Nature,* Harper and Row, San Francisco, 1980.
6. R. M. Zaner, The Phenomenon of Medicine: Of Hoaxes and Humor, in *The Culture of Biomedicine,* D. Heyward Brock and A. Harward (eds.), University of Delaware Press, Newark, Delaware, pp. 55-69, 1984.
7. D. Leder, A Tale of Two Bodies: The Cartesian Corpse and the Lived Body, in *The Body in Medical Thought and Practice,* Kluwer, Dordrecht, 1992.
8. M. Foucault, *The Birth of the Clinic,* Random House, New York, 1973.
9. E. J. Cassell, The Body of the Future, in *The Body in Medical Thought and Practice,* Kluwer, Dordrecht, 1992.
10. E. J. Cassell, *The Healer's Art,* J. B. Lippincott, Philadelphia, 1976.
11. H. Wulff, S. A. Pedersen, and R. Rosenberg, *Philosophy of Medicine,* Blackwell Scientific Publications, Oxford, pp. 30-45, 1990.
12. L. S. King, *The Medical World of the Eighteenth Century,* University of Chicago Press, Chicago, 1958.
13. G. L. Engel, How Much Longer Must Medicine's Science be Bounded by a Seventeenth Century World View?, in *The Task of Medicine,* K. L. White (ed.), The Henry J. Kaiser Family Foundation, Menlo Park, California, 1988.
14. H. Jonas, *The Phenomenon of Life,* Harper and Row, New York, 1966.
15. R. J. Carlson, *The End of Medicine,* John Wiley and Sons, New York, 1975.
16. D. E. Woolridge, *Mechanical Man: The Physical Basis of Intelligent Life,* McGraw-Hill, New York, pp. 9-18, 1968.
17. M. Hesse, *Revolutions and Reconstructions in the Philosophy of Science,* Indiana University Press, Bloomington, 1980.

18. M. Heidegger, The Question Concerning Technology, in *The Question Concerning Technology and Other Essays,* Harper and Row, New York, 1977.
19. R. Barthes, *New Critical Essays,* Hill and Wang, New York, pp. 23-39, 1980.
20. L. Foss and K. Rothenberg, *The Second Medical Revolution,* Shambhala, Boston, 1987.
21. J.-F. Lyotard, *The Postmodern Condition: A Report on Knowledge,* University of Minnesota Press, Minneapolis, 1984.
22. M. A. Schwartz and O. P. Wiggins, Scientific and Humanistic Medicine: A Theory of Clinical Methods, in *The Task of Medicine,* K. L. White (ed.), The Henry J. Kaiser Family Foundation, Menlo Park, California, 1988.
23. S. R. Bordo, *The Flight of Objectivity,* SUNY Press, Albany, 1987.
24. J. Habermas, *Knowledge and Human Interests,* Beacon Press, Boston, 1971.
25. R. Rorty, *Philosophy and the Mirror of Nature,* Princeton University Press, Princeton, 1979.
26. E. Straus, *Phenomenological Psychology,* Garland Publishing, New York, 1980.
27. P. Starr, *The Social Transformation of American Medicine,* Basic Books, New York, 1982.
28. M. Weber, *Economy and Society, Vol. I,* University of California Press, Berkeley, 1978.
29. S. Norell, Models of Causation of Epidemiology, in *Health, Disease, and Causal Explanation in Medicine,* L. Nordenfelt, B. Ingemar, and B. Lindahl (eds.), D. Reidel, Dordrecht, pp. 129-135, 1984.
30. E. Husserl, *The Crisis of European Sciences of Transcendental Phenomenology,* Northwestern University Press, Evanston, 1970.
31. R. Dubos, *The Mirage of Health,* Harper and Row, New York, 1959.
32. R. Dubos, *Man Adapting,* Yale University Press, New Haven, 1969.
33. E. L. Engel, *Psychological Development in Health and Disease,* W. B. Saunders, Philadelphia, 1962.
34. W. Stark, *The Fundamental Forms of Social Thought,* Fordham University Press, New York, 1963.
35. H. Strasser and S. C. Randall, *An Introduction to Theories of Social Change,* Routledge & Kegan Paul, London, 1981.
36. M. Mandelbaum, *History, Man, and Reason,* Johns Hopkins University Press, Baltimore, pp. 77-92, 1971.
37. P. Tillich, *Theology of Culture,* Oxford University Press, London, 1975.
38. J. Ellul, *The Technological Society,* Random House, New York, 1964.
39. J. W. Murphy and J. T. Pardeck, *The Computerization of Human Service Agencies,* Auburn House, New York, pp. 15-32, 1991.
40. H. L. Dreyfus and S. E. Dreyfus, *Mind Over Machine,* The Free Press, New York, pp. 101-121, 1986.

41. M. Foucault, *The Archaeology of Knowledge,* Routledge, London, 1989.
42. M. Weber, *The Protestant Ethic and the Spirit of Capitalism,* Scribner's, New York, 1958.
43. J.-F. Lyotard, *The Postmodern Condition: A Report on Knowledge,* University of Minnesota Press, Minneapolis, 1984.
44. E. Husserl, *The Crisis of European Sciences on Transcendental Phenomenology,* Northwestern University Press, Evanston, 1970.

CHAPTER 3

Major Components of the Biomedical Model

Freund and McGuire have argued that every understanding of the body is socially constructed [1]. There are cultural ideals *of* the body. No less important, however, are the philosophical developments *about* the body that are historically and culturally based. Emphasized in traditional Chinese medicine, for example, is an assortment of vital forces in the body (the *chi*), whose balance and manipulation bring about health. This vitalistic model is essentially non-material. In the West, by contrast, the body came to be understood in terms of biological science to be only material, and the scientific approach to medicine became overwhelmingly objective, reductionistic, and rational. The point is that whether in the East or West, these understandings of the body are equally cultural, and have evolved gradually. The concepts of biomedicine have formed over long periods of time, developing along the way a collection of integrated ideas that both explain and justify this view of medicine.

The end product of this process in the West is the "biomedical model." In this sense, scientific medicine is based on the physical and biological sciences. Some doctrines of the biomedical model more closely reflect the basic sciences (physics, chemistry, biology, and their derivative subspecialties), while others refer to the primary concern of scientific medicine, namely diseases located in the human body. Most important is that these beliefs hold together, thereby reinforcing one another and forming a coherent whole. There are five doctrines that make up the biomedical model. These are as follows: mind-body dualism, the mechanical analogy, physical reductionism, specific etiology and regimen and control.

Key at this juncture is that biomedicine is not necessarily a natural development. There is no *telos* guiding the growth of medicine, thereby guaranteeing the rationality of this discipline. Rather than the epitome of reason and objectivity, biomedicine is merely an option. Instead of exemplary, biomedicine represents a particular commitment to certain principles [2]. These considerations, as a result, are neither universal nor readily generalizable.

As is suggested in the previous chapter, a unique world-view encouraged the emergence of biomedicine, while the resulting culture supports the practices and procedures that are currently taken for granted as essential to medicine. What this means is that medicine is a symbolic enterprise. Biomedicine emerges from a unique form of discourse, and, in turn, the resulting body of values, beliefs, definitions, and commitments establishes the clearing in which physicians are currently expected to function. The value of biomedicine is thus a matter of convention—definition, ideology, and the exercise of influence—instead of dictated by its position on a mythical hierarchy of knowledge.

Because symbols must be interpreted before they gain any acceptance, the hegemony of biomedicine is challenged. Symbolism must be accepted before it is treated as real, and thus the universal stature of the biomedical model is called into question. Contrary to some critics, this realization does not signal that modern medicine is worthless. The medical advances over the past one hundred years, for example, should not be simply dismissed as fictional or unimportant. The point is that biomedicine is bound by interpretations of fact and history and can claim only limited relevance. Within a unique sphere the practice of biomedicine is entirely legitimate, but outside of this realm persons must be persuaded that this approach to illness has merit. Within a specific symbolic field biomedicine makes sense, and even represents the most effective means of treating those who are sick. Given the widespread acceptance of medicine today, this persuasion has been quite effective.

Nonetheless, the biomedical model is not exhaustive. For example, many social and cultural factors are omitted. Interventions are thus restrictive and directed mostly at physiological events. Yet biomedicine is not completely wrong, just narrow in scope. Biomedicine constitutes a partial truth that the medical establishment has tried to extend into almost every area. With good reason, such zealousness has been met with a lot of criticism.

What might be called the "culture of biomedicine" should be expanded only as far as its symbolic relevance allows [3]. For example, when a conceptualization of illness contains elements that extend beyond physiology, biomedicine should not dominate discussions about treatment. Clearly this impasse has been reached in the case of chronic disease, where definitions of social existence differ from those which delimit acute illness [4]. In fact, as will be discussed later, this disparity may constitute the most profound crisis yet to be faced by biomedicine.

What Eli Ginzberg calls the "curative bias" has blinded both the general citizenry and medical practitioners to these distinctions [5, p. 180]. In this sense, illness is presumed to have uniform qualities that underpin every malady; only surface discrepancies really exist. A basic structure is a part of every disease. Furthermore, the biomedical model plays an instrumental role in perpetuating this monolithic view of illness. The symbolic boundaries of illness are obscured due to the realism associated with biomedicine. Facts and not symbols, simply put, are the focus of most physicians. Indeed, symbols have no role in biomedicine. But the question remains: Is the symbolic universe of health and illness, not to mention truth and reality, encompassed by biomedicine?

As suggested by Fish, biomedicine is thoroughly political. Whoever thought that science would be linked to politics! After all, these positions are assumed traditionally to be anti-thetical. Yet when all truths are mediated by symbols, and thus reflect a perspective, the term political seems appropriate to describe this process [6, p. 8]. Like any political activity, however, biomedicine may have little appeal in some circles. This is not a fatal flaw, but simply a reality that should not be obscured behind labels such as reason, objectivity, value-freedom, and so forth. But ignoring this cipher of symbolism may prove to be deadly.

Why has the biomedical model been so widely accepted, given its limited scope? A partial answer is that this framework appears to be neat, concise, and helpful in dealing with many physical ailments. Nonetheless, this model is based on premises that are thoroughly shaky, and have begun to break down in practice. The biomedical model, accordingly, must be closely examined, particularly with regard to its theoretical underside.

MIND-BODY DUALISM

There is no way of avoiding the French mathematician and philosopher, Rene Descartes, in any discussion of the origins of medical science. As noted in Chapter 2, his work in the 1630s and 1640s laid the groundwork for the scientific method and for Western scientific medicine. The doctrine of mind-body dualism is attributed to him and provides the cornerstone that made scientific medicine possible.

Richard Zaner convincingly argues that Descartes is often misunderstood. Although Descartes asserts that one cannot accept the unity of the body and soul (mind) because they are different substances, in his discussions of clinical medicine he makes the point that the mind and body cannot be separated, because one affects the other in actual life. He warned a friend who was suffering from nose bleeding, for example, that he should avoid the use of strong substances such as mustard and vinegar, "as well as strong emotions."

Descartes pointed with pride to his eleven years of study in anatomy and physiology. In this context, Zaner continues, especially with respect to the dead body or cadaver, is where Descartes introduces mind-body dualism. The body can be studied as a system, in mechanical terms, once the mind or soul has left the body. One must remember that there were no MRI scanners, no x-ray machines, and not even any stethoscopes in 1630. Explorations of the body beyond exterior examinations required a cadaver. Accordingly, Descartes wrote that a medical examination of living patients should be conducted by "availing oneself only of life and ordinary conversations." Living persons should be treated differently than dead ones. Given this recommendation, dualism is not necessarily between mind and body, but between clinical and scientific medicine, or between the "lived" body and the dead body, the body with a mind and the inanimate body or cadaver.

Zaner believes that Descartes equivocated about the relationship between the body and soul. Nonetheless, the manner in which Descartes raised this issue set the stage for scientific medicine. The cadaver, in short, could be treated as a piece of meat. A corresponding step was easy to make, which identified a living person as an animated physiogamy. Yet in each case, physical features were simply obscured, according to Descartes, by mental phantasms. Separating these two elements was clearly not beyond the pale, but quite logical [7].

In fact, the medical scientists in the century following Descartes codified what today is understood as mind-body dualism, thus completely separating mind and body in the *living* patient. Thomas Boyle (1627-1691), Friedrich Hoffman (1660-1742) and La Mettrie (1709-1751) focused so much on the body that they even came to believe that the mind did not exist at all. By the early nineteenth century, the idea that the human body is the only proper subject of medical study had become orthodoxy. Nonetheless, Cartesian dualism, whether or not this idea came directly from Descartes, was seized by medicine as a means of organizing its view of the world, and is the cornerstone of the Western biomedical model. This schism of mind from body has led to the displacement of the patient as a person, as a result of encouraging that the body be examined as though it were a still-functioning corpse, devoid of mind or spirit. In Cassell's terms, dualism has substituted human pain for human suffering [8].

Zaner asserts that the triumph of Cartesian dualism resides most profoundly in the connection between pathology and diagnosis. The autopsy moves backward in the process from the death to its cause; the last chapter of existence is read first. By correlating pathological outcomes with presumed physiological causes, standards are established that allow the physician to make diagnoses that could be called "autopsies in advance." Interaction with the living person is not really necessary. Actually, such involvement gets in the way. A pure body, so to speak, provides a unique vantage point for summarizing the illness process. As a result of circumscribing a damaged component of a corpse, extrapolations can be made about the sequence of events that produced death. An alleged unadulterated foundation is available to justify this analysis. In light of dualism, the body is a fact that is stripped of mythology. The body is an Archimedean point, from which disease can be viewed with utmost clarity. Similar to Leibniz's pure monad, which reflects all perspectives, the body provides entree to the various facets of nature.

But the doctrine of mind-body dualism is a barrier to understanding the psychosocial and environmental components of medicine, including the placebo effect, the connection between stress and illness, the importance of social support, and, more generally, the relevance of life-style and issues pertaining to environmental health. The importance of the mind to most medical practitioners is, at root, a domain issue in medicine. Involving the mind in the science of the body can best be relegated to medical anthropology or behavioral medicine, so that medical science can stay close to its secure roots of biology, biochemistry, chemistry, physics, and their respective subspecialties. Although the dualism doctrine is no longer strictly adhered to, as in the case of behavioral medicine, the interaction between the mind and body is still considered to be peripheral to truly scientific medicine.

Medicine is so much more comfortable dealing with physiology than with extracorporeal phenomena, according to Foss and Rothenberg, that when confronted by an issue of mind/body interaction, medical scientists tend to fit the puzzle together by taking what they call a "hard science turn" [9]. For example, neuroscientists explain the effect of nonmaterial measures by translating them into their neurochemical correlates. They assert that a change in attitude is not affecting the patient, but that the neurochemicals released from the "body's own apothecary" are the source of any improvements. The focus is shifted quickly from the person who adopts the attitude to the body in which the physiological process occurs. This maneuver shifts the mind-body link to the brain-body connection, which is consistent with Cartesian dualism [10, p. 57].

The assumption of the physical nature of disease is rooted in materialism, but additionally this outlook is grounded in the scientific method that proposes to trust only the hardest, most reliable measures possible, and these are always physical. Foss and Rothenberg argue that this drift to the "hardest" data invariably focuses medical science on physiology, yet this refocusing is only possible by the separation of the mind and the wider society from the sick body. The result, of course, is that disease is located within the body.

In practice, what holds this cornerstone of the biomedical model in place is an attachment to biological science. Medical science is based on biology, and most biologists have tended to study biological systems, that is, the bodies of living or once-living creatures. These objects are material and not spiritual. Medical science is often viewed from the standpoint of the basic science curriculum of medical schools as the study of human biology. Engel asserts that the cultural authority of medical science is derived from the astonishing achievements of biology in the past century. This association, in part, explains the vast technological and financial resources that have been devoted to biomedicine [11]. Therefore, there is no incentive for medicine to abandon its roots any time soon.

But can the mind be separated from the body? If, at best, this is merely an analytical distinction, the current thrust of medicine would have to be redirected. The practice of medicine, in short, would have to become more patient or existentially centered. Modern theory and practice have illustrated that this shift is long overdue. More about this anti-dualistic tendency will be discussed in Chapter 6.

THE MECHANICAL ANALOGY

The second doctrine of the biomedical model descends directly from the writings of Descartes. After a careful reading of Descartes' work, Zaner concludes that at the end of the *Meditations* there is not a diad but a triad: "(1) what belongs to the mind considered 'in itself'; (2) what belongs to the body, and to body in general, considered 'in itself'; and (3) what belongs to the mind-body composite" [7, p. 118]. In the second case is where Descartes used the mechanical analogy, a fictional comparison with a clock or other mechanism. This, to Descartes, was the context of science, i.e., anatomy and physiology, and not necessarily clinical medicine. The third category, the mind-body composite, is what he used when discussing clinical medicine, and this context was surprisingly devoid of the machines that science uses as metaphors.

But even in Descartes' day, the heart was already being described as a mechanical pump. Harvey, in the early seventeenth century, discovered that blood circulates throughout the whole body, which represented a definite breakthrough that greatly impressed Descartes. Still, he had some reservations about the scope of this model. Yet physicians and philosophers who followed Descartes tended to take his mechanical characterizations more literally than he had intended, and to apply them in both scientific and clinical contexts.

Dossey assumes, perhaps too hastily, that the industrial revolution in Europe left an indelible impression on medical thought by way of the mechanical analogy, and that physicians were culturally trapped by their metaphors [12]. There is no doubt that there were new machines appearing regularly during this period and that public interest in mechanical engineering was widespread. Accordingly, the mechanical analogy was commonly and frequently used by nineteenth-century European physicians. The heart was a pump, and blood circulated in a manner similar to a hydraulic system; the lungs could be viewed as bellows, and the limbs perceived to operate by pulleys and levers. The question "How does it work?" was treated as an engineering inquiry and was in touch with the times. The mechanical analogy preceded the industrial revolution, however, and has roots more in biology than mechanical engineering. Nonetheless, the mechanical analogy served to concretize and formalize the study of the body. Ambiguity and speculation could be reduced about how living organisms functioned and managed to survive.

Dossey's interest in how persons become entrapped in metaphors is not altogether misplaced. In fact, the metaphors learned in medical schools are often carried over to a patient's bedside by professors in the later phases of medical education. Machines have interchangeable parts, if they are standardized. Moving from machine to body makes the assumption that human bodies are standardized, and thus this view tends to erode the understanding that each person has a unique background and unique variations in their bodies. Accordingly, physical examinations are regularly performed and a history taken that are consistent with making the leap to human interchangeability. Without a doubt, standardization has become the watchword of modern medicine. Zaner agrees with Dossey that when practicing physicians begin to think theoretically about patients, they are usually trapped by the accompanying metaphors. In this case, they find themselves before a physiological machine that needs to be repaired.

The well body is described as a fully functioning machine, and the sick body as a broken one. Similar to a machine, each part of the body contributes to the integrity of the whole. As a result of this portrayal, the search for the causes of a breakdown is facilitated. Mechanization is one of the "simplifying assumptions" that makes science possible [13, p. 62]. Simply put, the search for an easily identifiable organizing principle becomes viable. The problem comes when this imagery is taken for reality.

To understand the importance of the mechanical analogy to medical science, the reader must recall that a disease has been defined traditionally as a morbid state or process. Furthermore, this condition represents a deviation from norms that have measurable biological parameters. The concept of normality is central to modern medicine, and is often described as a "normal range" on various biological measures. Accordingly, departures from normality are diagnostic clues that the machine, or some part of it, is broken. Machines operate at an optimal level. These clues, additionally, often determine the intervention that will repair the machine and restore normal working order.

Hence, disease is viewed optimistically, as an eradicable physical condition. The diagnostic enterprise rests on the biological sciences, through which the biological "mechanisms" at work in normally functioning bodies are understood. This is not possible outside the language of the biophysical and physical sciences, which is presumed to be universal, objective, impersonal, ahistorical, acultural and, above all, material. The hope and goal of the biophysical sciences is to uncover the mechanisms of disease, and the physician uses this knowledge to intervene in the disease process and produce a cure, that is, to repair the machine [14, pp. 17-18]. The mechanical analogy, so conceived, is a picture of medical science's ultimate goal to understand fully the working of the normal human body and to restore its normal functioning.

For instance, Cassell has observed that the diagnosis of disease is normally based on the belief that each bodily function (as in kidney function) reflects a particular structure (as in the biochemistry and anatomy of the kidney). So when disease is noticed, the structure of an organ is the first place to look for a cause, microscopic or otherwise. Furthermore, the search for lesions such as tumors is predicated on this framework; lesions are understood to be structural abnormalities [8].

Dossey illustrates that the mechanical analogy continues to be updated as a consequence of new inventions. Today, for example, fascination with computers is often reflected in the analogies used by physicians, particularly neuropsychiatrists. Some human reactions are said to be "hard wired," entrenched in deep pathways called neural nets, and that is why many programs and systems within the body produce expected clinical outcomes. Like computers, brains are said to store information and access memory. The analogy comes down to the same conclusion that bodies are still machines, albeit ones that reflect the most recent technological developments.

This imagery has fed one obsession of the public. That is, medicine is imagined to be nothing more than a "technological fix." Pills, inoculations, gene splicing, and other "magic bullets" are thought to be available or just around the corner to cure every problem [15]. The most dire consequence of this belief is that disease is decontextualized, removed from history, and rendered impersonal. Medical practice, therefore, becomes very abstract. Technical remedies are matched with hypothetical bodies. Most problematic is that sometimes this match is effective, and citizens become further convinced that better medicine is synonymous with improved technology.

With regard to using a mechanical analogy, an important question is being asked in the philosophy of science. As theoretical physics moves away from the Newtonian theses that gave rise to the mechanistic perception of the world, and thus the mechanical view of the human body, one wonders whether mechanical metaphors will be gradually replaced by images generated by quantum mechanics? Foss and Rothenberg argue that such a paradigm shift is likely in the future because quantum theory allows self-organizing systems to be envisioned, such as the human body, that can adapt to environments where similar conditions may produce dissimilar products [9]. Human uniqueness would thus be elevated in importance.

The separation of structure and function in such models, and the overlapping of systems as they mutually influence one another, would be a radical break from the mechanical view. There is no doubt that change to include greater complexity in understanding human health will occur if quantum mechanics should produce a new analogy, and if that new imagery mirrors a reflexive or self-critical medical science. Clearly, quantum theory is merely another model, but one that represents a philosophy significantly different from the mechanical analogy. A quantum science, in short, is anti-dualistic, and thus amenable to the proposition that the mind and body are intermixed [16].

Other theories are available that make this theoretical move, such as the relativity, catastrophe and "boot strap" theses. What is significant about all of them is that facts are recognized to be shaped by a host of psychological, mathematical, and other constructs. Implied is that knowledge, including that related to the body, is not objective in the Cartesian sense. Facts, instead, are established by the nuances of conceptualization. The thrust of this maneuver for medicine is that the body is not an autonomous machine, but a conceptual scheme that can have a wide range of variations. If anything, complexity is the hallmark of quantum theory.

PHYSICAL REDUCTIONISM

The third part of the biomedical model is physical reductionism. Like dualism and the mechanical analogy, reductionism comes to the biomedical model from the nature of science. Reductionism is the attempt to understand the human body by studying its components and how they interrelate. Foss and Rothenberg outline the well known process whereby progressively more basic sciences attempt to explain phenomena in their own terms [9, pp. 62-64]. A disease is located, according to biomedicine, in a body. But, at least in principle, an organic disorder can be explained in ever smaller terms, which are proscribed by specialties such as pathophysiology, bacteriology, and histology. And these explanations can be further reduced by adopting the concepts, theories, and methods supplied by molecular biology, biological chemistry, and ultimately of physics. In fact, this is precisely the kind of thinking that has come to pervade medicine [13, pp. 43-60].

Reductionism, as it is used by scientists, may seem to be a straight-forward example of scientific imperialism, thus having more to do with academic arrogance and politics than with science. Although there is more than enough arrogance to go around in the scientific community, this conclusion is superficial and premature.

Physical reductionism is impossible to root out of biomedicine because this practice is epistemologically grounded in the scientific understanding of causation. In line with the mechanistic version of causality traditionally accepted by scientists, all bodily events also have determinate causes. Without this assumption, medical science, as we know it, would be impossible. As Hull writes:

> A type of explanation that originated in the study of purely physical phenomena has been extended to biological and social phenomena. All events are explained in terms of antecedent events organized in causal chains and networks, characterizable in terms of universal laws which make no reference to the causal efficaciousness of future events or higher levels of organization [17, p. 6].

Furthermore, reductionism is central to delineating these causal linkages. In order to specify explicitly the relationships among variables, complexity must be sacrificed. Identifying clear causal pathways requires that independent factors be joined *ad seriatim,* so that a neat sequence of events is established. Understanding data to exist in clusters, or constellations, violates this need for clarity. As a result, holism becomes an impediment to traditional scientific practice.

Science assumes an ordered universe, for otherwise the world could not be studied effectively, including the human body. In this connection, Foss and Rothenberg remind readers that levels of organization are assumed not to involve ontologically new entities beyond the elements of which they are comprised [9, pp. 104-113]. For example, molecules and only molecules are fundamental to cells. Assumptions supporting physical reductionism were at first approached tentatively in the history of science, and only later came to be viewed as scientific reality. They tend to give prior and thus greater status to the more basic "building blocks." And with regard to the organization of knowledge, physics is given primacy over chemistry, chemistry over biology, and biology over psychology. Therefore, the exclusion of the mind from medical considerations may be viewed as a particular case of physical reductionism. In the end, nonetheless, the discrete pieces of information essential for supporting causality are available; the mind, culture, and physical properties are sufficiently separated for clear delineations to be made among events.

Zucker makes this point clearly in his description of reductionism as a strategy in medicine:

> As a scientific strategy, reducing medicine to physiology means only that, where possible, research should take a certain bent toward molecular mechanisms. The presupposition of reduction in medicine is that all disease is physiology gone astray. Where there

is truly no physiological problem, there is no disease. . . . The ideal goal of reductionistic medicine would be diagnostics [and treatment] accomplished by a biochemical-biophysical survey of the patient's body. Ideally, psychological problems would be captured by this technique. It is part of the assumptions of reductionistic medicine that, at the very least, mental states have clinically useful physical correlates [18, pp. 149-150].

Given this commitment to reductionistic analysis, readers can begin to understand the discomfort and negative reactions of medical scientists to "alternative forms of medicine" that have their philosophical roots outside the paradigm of Western science. The same animosity is often noted when medical science confronts home-grown holistic medicine. The interaction between mind and body that is presumed by many of these holistic treatments is thought to violate the fundamental scientific understanding of causation. Specifically, scientists complain about the ambiguous concepts used in these approaches. Most physicians steeped in medical science are unable to justify the faith in mind-body interaction presupposed by these alternative medicines, because there is no epistemological basis for the anti-dualism that is often operative. Some "new age remedies," as they are sometimes called, presuppose an interrelationship of factors—such as the physical, cultural, spiritual, psychical, and even the cosmic—that is not given credence by traditionally trained physicians.

The doctrine of physical reductionism is at work in discussions of the genetic causes of disease. To be sure, reductionism would press toward genetic determinism [19]. Nobel Laureate Macfarlane Burnet is quoted by Zaner as asserting that medical science in this century has fostered the understanding that disease, injury, and handicap are preventable or treatable at the genetic level [20]. Only genetics remains to be seriously explored by medical science, and soon real progress will be made in treating these fundamental conditions. Burnet feels that nearly everything is determined by genetics, including human behavior and ultimately even war and evil, aging and death. In his view, there is simply no reality other than the genetic. Accordingly, genetic determinism is not an uncommon view these days. One result of holding such a belief is that persons are relieved of much responsibility for the current state of social affairs.

Particularly noteworthy is that the chemical tests conducted on blood and urine, for example, become more relevant than the patient's experience of illness or cultural considerations. The resulting data are usually quantified and easily inserted into explanatory models. But in the end, this search for simplicity becomes problematic; this version of Ocam's razor misconstrues the character of social life.

One maxim about social life is that society is complex. The interaction among factors is multivalent and, seemingly, ever expanding. In view of this variation, reductionism is counterproductive. Simplistic answers are given, in short, for very difficult problems. As a result, neat remedies are provided that are mostly, if not entirely, irrelevant. With regard to chronic illness, this simplicity is especially apparent. For as Strauss notes correctly, chronic disease is especially implicated in "organizational, social, economic, and social psychological" considerations [21, p. 5]. But most of these factors are envisioned to represent "soft data," according to proponents of the biomedical model, and are dismissed as tangential to making a diagnosis or prescribing a plan of treatment.

SPECIFIC ETIOLOGY

The fourth component of the biomedical model is an assumption about the causation of disease. This characteristic has come to be known as the doctrine of specific etiology. According to this principle, each disease state has a unique cause that can be discovered and attacked. The idea of a discrete cure, so central to heroic medical research, is grounded in this doctrine.

Historically, the doctrine of specific etiology is associated with the breakthrough research conducted by Louis Pasteur and Robert Koch in the 1860s and 1870s. These bacteriologists were able to isolate pathogens that caused some major infectious diseases, particularly tuberculosis. This rendition of causality was also strongly reinforced by germ theory and the invention of vaccines to attack the microbial origins of disease. These were important breakthroughs for medical science, because they substantially reinforced the cultural authority of physicians. Before this time, the efficacy of scientific medicine was not widely demonstrated or acknowledged. The search for "magic bullet" cures, when it motivates medical research, is promoted by this depiction of etiology.

The specific etiology thesis fits very comfortably within the framework of science, because this portrayal of causality is unilinear, concrete, and parsimonious. Spaeth and Barber have noted that such simple and ultimately artificial views of disease causation, however, affect adversely the way in which clinicians approach the concepts of disease and health [22]. Because medical students are taught to consider one disease per patient, as opposed to the intersection of several variables, a kind of parsimony drives research and treatment. Koch and Pasteur, in an artificial laboratory setting, could introduce one pathogen, a virulent microorganism, into a healthy animal and observe a clearcut sequence of events. Thus cause and effect were clear. Outside the laboratory, however, causation is rarely so tidy. Stated succinctly, some people exposed to microorganisms get sick and others do not. Intervening variables appear to be present that are not so easily circumscribed as a cause or effect.

Most disease processes involve the indirect influence of a complex set of factors, some predisposing, some precipitating, and some perpetuating, but all may be considered causes. In carefully controlled experiments, all of these can be eliminated except for the one infectious agent. Life, however, seldom imitates science. Unfortunately, however, the epistemology of science tends to mold and focus the clinician's view of life, whose diagnosis seeks to pinpoint *the* cause of disease and to treat it.

Exceptions to the assumptions of specific etiology are numerous. Diabetes can be treated by a therapeutic agent, insulin, but insulin does not cure diabetes. Furthermore, Dubos points out that human beings carry many dangerous microorganisms around in their intestines without infection [23]. Some other factor is apparently necessary to convert the infestation into disease. As evidence, he points out that cholera can be treated by hydrating patients and replacing electrolytes without any antimicrobial drug to combat the pathogen. The herpes simplex virus, acquired by most people during childhood, lies latent in their bodies for most of their lives, being activated from time to time by various physiological disturbances and appearing as fever blisters. The specific etiology doctrine is not helpful in explaining complex phenomena, such as those normally encountered in the life of the patient.

The point of these examples is to say that microorganisms, in themselves, do not necessarily cause disease. If this were the case, a one-to-one correlation would exist between the presence of a pathogen and the onset of illness. Obviously, illness does not occur in this way. Stress and other cultural considerations, for instance, mediate the pathogen-disease relationship and add complexity to this causal association. Understanding the physiological impact of a germ or virus, accordingly, may have little to do with predicting the likelihood of a person becoming sick. The sequence of precipitating events are not this simple.

As an important dimension of the biomedical model, the view that a disease has a specific cause that can be cured keeps the focus of research, diagnosis, and treatment on the human body, as opposed to the contributing or participating factors outside of physiology. No one dies directly from smoking or smog, but these factors can clearly contribute to disease outcomes. And by focusing on specific etiology attention is diverted away from issues of health promotion or disease prevention, and thus this viewpoint tends to depreciate public health approaches to industrial and environmental medicine.

Finally, the principle of specific etiology fits neatly into the infectious disease model. Infectious diseases, however, have declined in importance, except for AIDS. Single causes and cures are a key part of how the spread of infections are studied. but such scientific parsimony is increasingly rare in the clinical world. Each clinical decision can involve so many judgments of facts and values that, in Dubos' words, "medicine in its highest form will continue to remain an art," medical science not withstanding [23, pp. 97-102].

REGIMEN AND CONTROL

The fifth aspect of the biomedical model asserts that the body is the appropriate locus of regimen and control. This principal is a logical corollary of physical reductionism. If disease exists in the body, then the body would be the appropriate locus of treatment. Specific etiology concerns discovery and diagnosis; regimen and control concern the treatment that follows from a diagnosis.

The hospital was meant to isolate the patient so that the doctor could exercise more control in both diagnosis and treatment. In a hospital, the physician could, in effect, hold other variables constant when searching for a cause and applying a treatment for a disease. Treatment, therefore, is modeled after the scientific method, just as is the diagnostic work done on the front end.

Moving down the decision tree to a diagnostic conclusion is easier when patients are in the hospital, rather than in their communities. Despite what the medical model has to say, the patient is not a passive partner in the therapeutic relationship. What patients believe about their condition will encourage them to modify or even nullify the cogent scientifically derived or reasonably concluded answers of a physician. If the mind could just be separated from the body, along with a host of other factors, then the body could be objectively treated. The biomedical model works better in the laboratory than in the daily life of the patient. Compliance with regimen and control requires a great deal of the patient. Specifically, patients must believe in the skill and power of the healer and the efficacy of his or her medications and procedures. Additionally, they must understand and be willing to follow directions.

For this reason, patients are now understood to fare better when treated in their communities. In fact, during the 1960s policies were made that mandated treatment be undertaken in the "least restrictive environment" [24]. Nonetheless, many physicians rejected this philosophy, due to the uncertainties that would be interjected into the treatment setting. The influence of non-professionals, environmental exigencies, and other sources of variance could not be controlled. Under such conditions, physicians believed that treatment would be ineffective, and possibly harmful and refused to be implicated in this community-based strategy. Their commitment to science, they argued, was incompatible with this project.

Biomedically inspired regimen and control, however, are very intensive. Patients are removed from support groups, placed in a sterile environment, monitored and probed, and evaluated by scientific instruments. Yet such treatment has proven to be harmful to patients; they often become disoriented, depressed, and unresponsive to help [25]. A type of institutionalized illness often sets in, whereby patients become fully dysfunctional.

When a physician listens only to the body and not to the person's experience of illness and what is going on in the person's life, the patient, who is a person, is less likely to comply with the regimen prescribed by the physician. At this point, the biomedical model breaks down. Out-patient treatment, for example, is especially difficult within the parameters of biomedicine. This strategy involves cultural factors that cannot be neatly circumscribed. Nonetheless, chronic illness is addressed mostly on an out-patient basis. Here again, the treatment of chronic problems runs into trouble.

CONCLUSION

The body, in itself, apart from mind or culture, is singled out as the location of disease; in that body there are disease mechanisms at work that the doctor can alter to affect a cure. These factors, moreover, are understood to reside at the more basic biophysical levels, so that *the* cause can be identified and a treatment regimen designed for a patient that will be successful. That is the biomedical model in a nutshell.

The way that the model is worked out in the therapeutic relationship is instructive. Patients are less likely to be asked how they feel than where they hurt, thus keeping the focus always on the body. Once a complaint is located, testing begins that provides evidence for several alternative diagnostic hypotheses. One variable after another is eliminated by mixing and matching the data points, until a particular cause is identified that makes sense within a functional (mechanistic) framework. The patient is then given medicine to cure the disease or surgery is recommended to remove the diseased tissue. Given this *modus operandi,* the biomedical model works best in the presence of acute illness that can be readily encompassed and cured.

The situation for the clinical practitioner, however, is not as simple and easy as advocates of the biomedical model seem to think. In identifying a problem, the physician is more likely to focus on classificatory patterns than the individual patient, thus transforming a unique individual into a specimen. When the hypothesized problem is diagnosed, the patient is labeled and treated accordingly. But classifying the pathological mechanism is easy compared to understanding how this pathogen is working in an individual, living patient who is not an isolated body, but also has a mind and is adapted (or maladapted) to a complex social and physical environment. Clearly, the biomedical model is elegant in its simplicity, as compared to dealing with the actual problems of a sick patient.

This discussion of the biomedical model has remained at the theoretical level. Perhaps a better way to understand how philosophy has shaped medical practice is to examine briefly the rise of scientific medicine, paying particular attention to the development of medical technology. In this regard, the actual impact of certain concepts can be appreciated.

What should be noticed in the following chapter is the attempt that has been made to bring physicians into *direct* contact with the causes of diseases. Direct or unencumbered observation has been thought to be essential to the discovery of facts. Of course, this ability is considered to be a key part of science and biomedicine. But human observational abilities are variable and often inaccurate. Therefore, overcoming the weaknesses of perception has been an obsession throughout the history of modern medicine.

REFERENCES

1. P. E. S. Freund and M. B. McGuire, *Health, Illness, and the Social Body: A Critical Sociology,* Prentice Hall, Englewood Cliffs, New Jersey, 1991.
2. K. Racevskis, *Postmodernism and the Search for Enlightenment,* University Press of Virginia, Charlottesville, pp. 65-77, 1993.
3. D. H. Brock and A. Harward (eds.), *The Cultural of Biomedicine,* University of Delaware Press, Newark, 1984.
4. D. M. Fox, *Power and Illness,* University of California Press, Berkeley, 1993.
5. E. Ginzberg, *A Pattern for Hospital Care,* Columbia University Press, New York, 1949.
6. S. Fish, *There's No Such Thing as Free Speech,* Oxford University Press, New York, 1994.
7. R. Zaner, *Ethics and the Clinical Encounter,* Prentice Hall, Englewood Cliffs, New Jersey, 1988.
8. E. J. Cassell, *The Nature of Suffering and the Goals of Medicine,* Oxford University Press, New York, 1991.
9. L. Foss and K. Rothenberg, *The Second Medical Revolution: From Biomedicine to Infomedicine,* Shambhala, Boston, 1987.
10. A. Weil, *Health and Healing,* Houghton Mifflin, Boston, 1983.
11. G. L. Engel, The Need for a New Medical Model: A Challenge for Biomedicine, Science, 196, 1977.
12. L. Dossey, *Meaning and Medicine: Lessons from a Doctor's Tales of Breakthrough and Healing,* Bantam Books, New York, 1991.
13. M. R. Werbach, *Third Line Medicine,* Arkana, New York, 1986.
14. J. D. Beasley, *The Betrayal of Health,* Random House, New York, 1991.
15. T. Kaptchuk and M. Croucher, *The Healing Arts,* Summit Books, New York, pp. 77-89, 1987.
16. D. Zohar, *The Quantum Self,* Bloomsbury Publishing, London, 1990.
17. D. Hull, Reduction and Genetics, *Journal of Medicine and Philosophy, 6,* 1981.
18. A. Zucker, Holism and Reductionism: A View from Genetics, *Journal of Medicine and Philosophy, 6,* 1981.
19. A. Etzioni, Health Care and Self-care: The Genetic Fix, in *Where Medicine Fails,* Anselm L. Strauss (ed.), Transaction Books, New Brunswick, New Jersey, pp. 189-201, 1979.
20. M. Burnet, *Endurance of Life: The Implications of Genetics for Human Life,* Cambridge University Press, London, 1978.
21. A. L. Strauss, Introduction, in *Where Medicine Fails,* Transaction Books, New Brunswick, New Jersey, 1979.
22. G. L. Spaeth and G. W. Barber, Homocystinuria and the Passing of the One Gene-one Enzyme Concept of Disease, *Journal of Medicine and Philosophy, 5,* 1980.

23. R. Dubos, *Mirage of Health: Utopias, Progress, and Biological Change,* Doubleday and Company, Inc., Garden City, 1959.
24. W. A. Vega and J. W. Murphy, *Culture and the Restructuring of Community Mental Health,* Greenwood Press, Westport, Connecticut, pp. 1-20, 1990.
25. J. K. Wing and G. Brown, *Institutionalism and Schizophrenia,* Oxford University Press, Oxford, 1978.

CHAPTER
4

The Rise of Scientific Medicine

Scientific medicine developed as a result of adopting and applying science to medical concerns. Once science was accepted culturally, the stage was set for medicine to move into a new arena. In short, science came first. Also, although science, in its pure form, has always been primarily concerned with understanding the measurable (i.e., physical) world, the focus of scientists is on basic processes and mechanisms, and not necessarily the application of scientific principles to human goals such as health or welfare. Bio-physical science found its major applications in medicine, much as physics found its primary application in engineering. Indeed, the science courses in medical schools are usually taught by instructors whose ID tags carry a Ph.D. rather than an M.D. after their names.

The theory that health came from a harmony or balance of the four fluids (humors) in the body—blood, mucus, yellow bile, and black bile—dominated Western medicine for most of its early history. Zaner explains that those physicians who based their understanding of medicine on humoral theories took symptoms as signs of invisible inner bodily events, i.e., humoral imbalances [1]. Physicians who believed in these dogmas had to understand these symptoms and make diagnoses based on them. The treatment they prescribed, however, was aimed not at the symptoms but at restoring balance within the body. For example, they would draw blood from the different parts of the body to restore harmony, depending on how certain symptoms were interpreted. The instrument for drawing blood was the "lancet," a tool that was adopted as the name of the leading medical journal in England today. Additionally, leeches could be found often in apothecaries in the United States into the nineteenth century, for the purpose of bleeding a person.

The point is that physicians of earlier centuries did not ignore the body's curative and restorative powers. Instead, Zaner argues that "empiric" tendencies were also present in "pre-scientific" medicine; interventions were not guided solely and always by dogma [1, pp. 137-140]. Taking detailed histories of illness experiences and the preceding events, and skillfully encouraging the body to heal itself, has a long history before science came to dominate medicine. These practices served historically and theoretically as a background for homeopathy, which is the type of medicine that was adopted widely in Western Europe and the United States in the eighteenth and nineteenth centuries. Physicians often combined dogmatic and empiric approaches, and achieved enough success to stay in business and occasionally to earn acclaim as skilled healers.

Dogmatic physicians, however, took the more heroic approach to medicine, using forceful treatments to affect immediate cures, such as blood-letting, or prescribing strong medicines to induce vomiting or bowel evacuation. The gentler and slower cures were associated with the empiricists and herbalists. In this sense, the lineage of scientific medicine, Zaner argues, leads directly to the dogmatics. But in general, Foucault contends that the rise of scientific medicine occurred when physicians decided to return to the "modest but effecting level of the perceived" [2, p. xii]. Empirical regularities, in other words, gradually became the focus of attention.

SCIENTIFIC DISEASE THEORY

Rather credits Plato with the idea that symptoms are not the reflection of invisible causes, as the dogmatists believed [3]. Instead, patterns of symptoms correspond to specific disease entities, a point that is taken as a truism today. The Greeks, writes Sigerist, believed that "disease is a natural process, not basically different from physiological processes" [4, p. 11]. Reiser resumes this story with Thomas Sydenham, a seventeenth-century English physician who asserted that recurring patterns of symptoms could be used to identify the patient's specific disease.[1] In some ways, his diagnostic perspective was similar to Greek dogmatic physicians, who saw symptoms as clues that point to

---

[1] This chapter draws heavily upon Reiser's material, generally summarizing and following the outline of his book. His discussion is the best single analysis of the rise of medical technology.

the particular unseen humoral imbalance in the patient's body. Nonetheless, Sydenham became known for recommending that physicians go to a patient's bedside, if they want to learn about illness. For symptoms, writes Reiser, "indicate[d] any departure from good health" [5, p. 1]. In short, symptoms are real and empirical. And because they exist in tissues, the body became the locus of the search for disease [6, p. 12].

A number of eighteenth-century physicians continued in Sydenham's footsteps, primarily using pre-existing descriptive data to classify diseases. Prominent among these was a physician-botanist of the period, Francoise Boissier de Sauvages, who in 1731 offered a detailed classificatory scheme. Thirty years later his classification had grown to include 2,400 species of diseases, grouped into ten classes, forty orders, and 295 genera. Is there any doubt that medicine was modeling itself after natural science? Diseases were viewed to be like flora. William Cullen, professor of medicine at Edinburgh, in his 1769 treatise, reduced and recodified earlier classifications. He encouraged the search for "pathognomonic" symptoms, which occurred in clusters and were associated regularly with particular diseases.

Clearly medicine was adopting Bichat's advice to pay attention to observable events; "look and see" is what he used to say. There was much to be gained by opening a few bodies and finding the diseased point that underpins all symptoms. Accordingly, the signs provided by symptoms could be interpreted without any reference to mythology, or any other ethereal considerations [4, p. 2].

Disease theory developed rapidly in the early decades of the nineteenth century in France [7]. The classification of diseases was a conscious effort to introduce science into medicine. Having a universal classificatory scheme was viewed as essential for securing common understanding among doctors. Once diseases, which were viewed ontologically as "things," were defined and consensus was gained on these definitions, the search for their causes, or etiology, could proceed apace.

Most modern scientists base their classifications on diseases found in living patients. They are not interested in classifications derived from autopsies, because a disease cannot be understood divorced from the disease process. And this process, of course, comes to a halt when death occurs.

But the observation of living persons is difficult. Their dynamic nature is hard to control, and thus observations may be compromised by various extraneous, or non-empirical elements. Nonetheless, to truly understand disease requires that illness be captured *in vivo*.

Otherwise, extrapolations will be necessary that are speculative. The *Körper,* however, is easy to constrain and observe. But investigating live persons remains the ideal.

PATHOLOGICAL ANATOMY AND
CARTESIAN DUALISM

This is an important point, because by the eighteenth century doctors were beginning to rely heavily on autopsies to supply their understanding of disease. To be sure, the origins of human anatomy go back to much earlier times. Reiser traces this history, beginning with Galen, a second-century physician, who attempted to describe the organs of human bodies by comparing them with those present in dissected animals, particularly the Barbary ape. Orthodox understandings of anatomy were based on Galen's observations for over a century. In point of fact, legal proceedings during the late Middle Ages sometimes ordered dead bodies to be opened in search for evidence of poisoning, when foul play was suspected.

Vesalius, professor at Padua in the 1540s, urged physicians to observe directly the anatomy, instead of relying solely on textbook knowledge. Vesalius' attitude was scientific in the sense that he was exploring the natural world to find facts. In doing so, he found that Galen had been wrong at many points where the anatomy of apes and humans differed. Furthermore, the step from normal to pathological anatomy was revealed to be a small one. The idea also became clear that an observation made by one student can be verified by other students, and on the bases of these comparative studies a body of verified knowledge about disease can be systematically developed. In 1554, for example, Frenchman Jean Fernel examined lesions (structural abnormalities) in cadavers, but talked about them in terms of the symptoms of diseases. By the time that Sydenham was writing in England about disease histories and disease species, collections of autopsy data were being published that were filled with clinical descriptions and findings. The result was a more comprehensive and concrete picture of disease, along with the most propitious points for introducing interventions. To many observers, progress was being made in terms of accumulating a reliable stock of medical knowledge.

According to Zaner, a major turning point in the study of pathological anatomy and in medical science came in 1761 when Giovani Morgagni's treatise, *The Seats and Causes of Diseases Investigated by Anatomy,* appeared [8]. He was the first to correlate observations made during an autopsy with the clinical symptoms reported before the death of *the same patient*. These clinico-pathological correlations allowed physicians to predict the disease outcome from the symptoms observed in living patients. Morgagni used the autopsy to "explain" the symptoms, thus projecting backward in time. At the time, however, most physicians were still concentrating on treating symptoms only. According to Reiser, disease was not generally understood to be localized in the organism. But Morgagni was able to show the "footprints left by disease" in the body, thereby helping physicians to verify their judgments. This was a turning point in body-centered medicine, and in support of the emerging biomedical model.

The location of lesions within the organs of the body became progressively refined after Morgagni. The French physician, Xavier Bichat, made one such major step in 1801 when he showed that the entire organ often was not diseased. Lesions occurred in grossly visible biological substances that he called "tissues," which he went on to classify in twenty-one types. Tissues, he argued, are the building blocks of organs. The contribution of Bichat to the biomedical model, according to Zaner, is found in his insistence that the history of a disease is not important, and that the patient's observations and reports are irrelevant and to be ignored [1, pp. 132-134]. With Bichat, symptoms were understood to originate from the lesion. As a result, the patient was separated from his or her body completely. Arney and Bergen refer to this development as "the disappearance of the experiencing person" [6, pp. 9-28].

Cartesian dualism had taken hold and become the hallmark of the nineteenth-century medical scientist. This attitude toward the body, however, would be refined further in the history of Western medicine. But by adopting the theory of localized pathology, Reiser argues, the physician was moving closer to a surgeon's view of disease, which had always been body-centered. Pathological anatomy, therefore, encouraged the increasing convergence of medicine and surgery in the 1800s.

THE PHYSICAL EXAMINATION

The physical examination, as it is experienced today, evolved from obscure origins early in the last century. As previously discussed, examining the insides of dead bodies by physicians, however, preceded the investigation of living ones by a very long while. The historical record reveals that pathological anatomy was well established before physicians began listening to the body's internal signs. Nevertheless, Reiser states that in 1761, the same year that Morgagni's important treatise appeared, a Viennese physician, Leopold Auenbrugger, published a monograph in which he described a method of examination he called "percussion" [5, pp. 20-22]. The general procedure is well known to those who thump watermelons to determine their degree of ripeness. Percussion was a method of listening to the sounds reflected from the inside of a living body. The method was not readily accepted, however, because these sounds were difficult to describe verbally, so that those who read the descriptions would know which echoes were relevant. Observations were not direct, and thus extrapolations had to be made from vague sounds. Also, the application of manual methods seemed beneath the dignity of many physicians, who saw themselves as word-oriented rather than touch-oriented. Consequently, percussion as a diagnostic technique was not widely adopted at that time.

The decades between 1800 and 1830 mark the shift away from philosophically-based classical medicine to scientifically-based clinical medicine. Because of new technical devices, observations were allegedly not obscured by theory, words, or any other mode of subjectivity [9, pp. 108-111]. Perhaps better than any other event, the invention of the first crude stethoscope by a young French physician Rene Laennec in 1816 symbolizes the shift in perspective. Starr observed that before Laennec doctors observed patients but now they *examined* them [10]. Physicians had put their ear to the chest of patients before 1816, but the strait, wooden stethoscope was much more convenient, tasteful, and allowed physicians to hear the chest sounds of even obese patients. Laennec spent much of his career promoting the stethoscope. Reiser reports that he was very skeptical of the outward signs of chest disease, i.e., coughing, expectorating, and shortness of breath, and that he distrusted patient narratives. The stethoscope localized pathology in a way that outward signs or verbal descriptions could not. The physician heard with his own ear more accurate signs, "harder" data, than could be supplied by the accounts of patients [11, p. 220]. An interesting aside, however, is that the older technique of percussion gained greater merit when combined with a stethoscope.

But the stethoscope was not accepted immediately. Laennec demonstrated that the sounds he heard did predict the lesions revealed in autopsies. And as might be expected, this test increased the instrument's acceptance. The idea of "seeing" a defective physical structure by listening to the body captured the imagination of physicians, and the leap forward in the diagnosis of chest diseases seemed to be a major one, indeed. The physical examination of patients, using the stethoscope, seemed to bring physicians closer to the dream of basing their practice on unencumbered observations. Chest disease would no longer be hidden from physicians. In a sense, the physician could see inside patients before their deaths. The model of chest disease deduced from sounds, and confirmed by autopsy, came to replace other models that had been based on patient reports and crude observations. Still, this new mode of listening was not very sophisticated. Nonetheless the binaural tube stethoscope, which today symbolizes clinical medicine, did not displace the stick version until the last decade of the nineteenth century.

As scientific medicine developed into the mid-1800s, doctors paid more attention to physiological markers. To stethoscopes were added instruments that helped physicians literally to look inside the body. Ophthalmoscopes, for observing the retina of the eye, and laryngoscopes, for scanning the throat, and the metal speculum, for peering into the vagina, all strengthened the physician's sensory powers when conducting clinical examinations. In the process, however, the personal side of medicine became increasingly less relevant [12, p. 46]. Technology became the cipher of health.

Some critics sill argued that the physical examination did not provide the kind of evidence that best promoted science, because the individual physician's observations of signs were made in isolation. Contrary to this mode of study, science requires consensus based on objective and shared evidence. The subjective reports of patients were being rejected as evidence; the uncorroborated reports of the physician-observers were also being disputed by other physicians. One great invention in the middle of the nineteenth century enabled physicians to compare judgments on the same physical evidence, thereby accelerating the evolution of scientific medicine. This device was the camera.

MEDICAL PHOTOGRAPHY

After all, as reported by writers such as Roland Barthes, most of the public continues to believe that cameras simply reflect reality [13]. When this technology was first invented, naive realism was mostly unquestioned. Through the use of the camera, unadulterated facts could finally be depicted. Reiser argues that photography transformed medicine by recasting and standardizing the physician's images of disease. Pictures captured events in operating theaters, autopsy rooms, and hospital wards. Accordingly, medical students studied photographs to sharpen their powers of clinical observation. Even more important, the fact that physicians were learning to visualize and agree on the exterior representations of pathology, prepared them to accept x-ray images of the body's interior.

In 1895 when Wilhelm Roentgen, a physics professor at the University of Wurzgburg in Bavaria, found that cathode rats could variably penetrate solids according to their density, and that these images could be captured on photographic plates, the world changed for scientific medicine [9, pp. 408-417]. A bony portrait of his wife's hand was the first x-ray of a human being. Few previous diagnostic discoveries had stirred so much interest. The x-ray picture represented a quantum leap forward in the physician's ability to observe the human body. For example, bones could be set and bullets extracted more easily than in the past. Shadow portraits of bones, gall and kidney stones, and internal organs showed physicians the new territory that lay before them. In only five years, by 1900, x-rays were being used also in the courts in malpractice suits, thus evoking some concern in the medical profession.

From the standpoint of the biomedical world, the x-ray was a critical turning point. Physicians needed the patient before them to use the other visualization tools, including the stethoscope. Those who used the photograph, and particularly the x-ray, could debate the diagnosis of patients, directly from physical evidence, without requiring them to be present. The body was thereby separated from the person much more profoundly than ever before. From the perspective of science, the photograph provided an objective and permanent record that transcended both memory and subjective impression. Hence a new and more secure path to medical truth had been furnished, according to the proponents of scientific medicine.

A third type of photography, photomicrography, also sped up the evolution of medical science. This practice gave considerable support to several doctrines of the biomedical model, most notably those of physical reductionism and specific etiology. The history of microscopy has been summarized nicely by Reiser [5, pp. 87-90]. Magnifiers had been used for years to study physical phenomena too small to be seen clearly by the unaided eye. For example, the English scholar, Roger Bacon, used convex lenses to magnify images as early as the thirteenth century. During the mid-1600s, the most notable early microscopists were describing the structure of the lungs, spleen, and kidney, and examining the early stages of animal embryo development. Further, the capillaries that connect arteries to veins were described by the Italian physician Marcello Malpighi, thereby supporting the early theories of the blood's circulation. And Robert Hook of England, in 1665, was the first to describe the biological structure of cells. The visual distortion created by the lenses of the time, however, made the microscope a difficult and unreliable scientific instrument. Not until 1829 did Joseph Jackson Lister, an English wine merchant, find a way to reduce lens distortion from 19 percent to 3 percent, thus making the microscope a reliable window into the cellular world.

After 1829, the microscope became an increasingly valuable tool of medical science [14, p. 91]. Bichat, since the opening days of the century, had preached the importance of tissue destruction in gross anatomy. Now microscopes were available to examine the tissue's elementary constituents. Cancer tumors could thus be brought into view and their microstructure classified.

Inevitably cellular pathology would become a field of study in its own right and make a claim to scientific knowledge of the body. Reiser reports that the process of physical reductionism was by this time evident in looking for the source of disease at the cellular level [5, pp. 78-79]. Rudolf Virchow's treatise, *Cellular Pathology,* was published in 1858, and in this book he insisted that the cell is the only proper locus for studying the fundamentals of life. This point of view implies that patients are little more than a mosaic of cells and other micro-elements.

But microscopic analysis did not end with the study of cells. Actually, this was only the beginning. Soon every disease was thought to have a micro-cause, and the search was underway for these minute entities. Attention was suddenly directed to germs, viruses, and other minute organisms.

The study of microorganisms as causal agents of infectious diseases is associated with Louis Pasteur of France and Robert Koch of Germany [15]. Microorganisms could not have been identified without the microscope. But given the availability of this technology, bacteriology provided the most dramatic breakthroughs of medical science during the nineteenth century, a time when many useful discoveries were made. Tuberculosis was responsible for approximately every seventh death in Europe when Koch discovered the tubercle bacillus and an inoculation for this disease in 1882. No medical discovery could have focused more attention on the microscope, bacteriology, and cellular medicine. This breakthrough introduced to the lay public a view of physiological disorder that came to be called "germ theory," and raised the hope that medical science could cure most maladies by making further discoveries at the cellular level. The leverage that such success gave to biomedical science was enormous, and for many physicians microorganisms became the paramount diagnostic signs. They reasoned that addressing the secondary effects of disease is unimportant, if the actual agent of disease can be directly confronted. Accordingly, physicians were encouraged to become "microbe hunters" and strategies were devised to identify, isolate, and destroy these almost invisible sources of disease [16].

Germs came to be seen as *the* cause of disease. In line with this new orientation, the public health movement in Europe that aimed to improve sanitation gained speed. The process of killing bacteria by raising the temperature of milk, now known as pasteurization, was named for Louis Pasteur, and a popular mouth wash was later named for Joseph Lister the inventor of antiseptic surgery. Lister, incidentally, was the son of the English wine merchant who perfected the microscope [11, pp. 351-354]. Despite the fact that bacteriology could not explain the variability of resistance to infection among human beings, microorganisms were thought to supply a realistic view of disease causation.

The microscope became the symbolic logo of medical research, just as the stethoscope had become for clinical medicine. Indeed, photographs of medical scientists by the turn of the twentieth century very often showed them sitting at a microscope. The microscope, due to the discoveries that it afforded, finally wedded clinical medicine and science. Examinations with the microscope could take place in the absence of the tissue donor, thereby separating completely the patient from the doctor during diagnosis. In this regard, the x-ray and the microscope were instrumental in reinforcing the principle of value-neutrality, and the belief that human observations could be flawless.

STANDARDIZED MEASURES OF PHYSICAL FUNCTIONING

From the time of Morgagni and Bichat, the clinico-pathological correlation had been the major approach to identifying disease. Theory and practice, simply put, were not clearly associated, because observations were thought to be replete with human error and not trustworthy. A reappraisal of this approach began with the technology that allowed the examiner to hear or see the inside of the living patient by using the stethoscope and the x-ray. Reiser discusses the many other techniques, tools, and machines which were added during the nineteenth century, thereby quantifying essential bodily functions, such as breathing, the circulation of the blood, and temperature, for use in rendering a diagnosis [5, pp. 91-121]. To photographs were added graphs and charts, which illustrated objective physical signs that could vary from the norm of health and thereby indicate a disease state. To the body's architecture, understood through anatomy, was added what seemed to be objective measures of function. The focus was thus directed to the living patient, while the study of pathology was standardized. Hence comparative analysis was greatly improved.

For example, counting the pulse, a very old technique, eventually became a standardized technique for studying blood circulation. In 1860, the beat of a pulse could be translated into a visual form—a line drawn on paper—by using a sphygmometer. Yet the high hopes for diagnoses raised by the inventors of these machines eventually faltered, because of the many unresolved issues related to standardized measurements. Simply put, conceptualization and measurement are not antipodes, and thus assessments are never direct but mediated by cognition and always partial. The attempt at standardization, therefore, failed to produce unadulterated vision. Nonetheless, the work of Samuel von Basch, in 1876, which attempted to measure high blood pressure, paid off and laid the foundation for Riva-Rocci's (1896) air-filled cuff and rubber bulb pump that is still used today.

Additionally, in 1887, Augustus Waller noticed that the electrical currents generated by the human heart that could be detected by surface measures. And in 1901, Willem Einthoven devised a way of measuring these impulses and the electrocardiograph was invented. After 1918 when researchers demonstrated that coronary artery blockage produced specific changes in the patient's electrocardiograph, this device became a major diagnostic tool.

Fever was a sign of disease among early Greek physicians. And Galileo measured body heat crudely in 1593. However, during the seventeenth and eighteenth centuries attempts to make thermometers failed, because of measurement issues related to atmospheric pressure, the type of fluid used, and the scale adopted. Finally, mercury was agreed on because this semi-fluid was heavy enough to offset atmospheric pressure, while Fahrenheit's scale was adopted over other contenders. By 1860, the thermometer had become generally accepted as a valuable device for measuring body temperature in an objective way.

Reiser summarizes these developments, saying that the

> conversion of physiological signals generated by respiration, circulation and heat production into graphs and numbers, allowed physicians to obtain clear and accurate records; to preserve these signals from the limitations of private analysis—necessary when they were individually monitored by the natural senses—and open them to group inquiry; to make them objective and to invest them with unambiguous meanings that were evident to all physicians [5, p. 121].

More germane to this chapter, these developments also have arisen from and were reinforced by the biomedical model. They keep the focus on the body, as a consequence of translating its functions into mechanistic terms. Further, these standardized measures reinforce the illusion that the body is a predictable and closed physical system that operates only by natural law, and can be understood adequately only in this way. Most proponents of science argue that quantification is necessary for facts to be discovered and sound judgments made. To the extent that medical research and clinical practice overlap and inform one another, the emphasis placed on quantification will probably only intensify.

By the early 1900s, standardized rates and actuarial tables for comparing a patient to populations had been introduced to help physicians make objective judgments, based on the idea of normality. Eye charts, weight-height tables, and IQ tests are examples of the inventions of this period. In each case, normalcy is associated with objective criteria that are devoid of the uncertainty associated with subjectivity. Normal and abnormal, as dichotomous concepts, came to reign supreme in clinical medicine and served to guide both diagnostic and treatment decisions. But as Foucault points out, the result is that health is overlooked because of this concern for normalcy. His point is that normalcy has nothing to do, necessarily, with how individuals feel and view themselves [2, p. 35]. Health is more of a holistic matter than normalcy.

Removing disease from its location in the interactive person, to a physical body, may have been the first order reduction envisioned in mind-body dualism. But this was hardly the end, for the search for disease has been reduced to more and more basic levels of the physical world. The second major step along this path was the effective use of photography, the microscope, and other technical aids in medicine, which opened the door to the cellular world and placed the study of disease squarely in the domain of the biological sciences. But there is a third level of reduction that can be identified with the nineteenth and early twentieth centuries in the growth of scientific medicine. This is the advent of chemistry and the growth of diagnostic laboratories.

MEDICAL CHEMISTRY AND DIAGNOSTIC LABS

The visible features of urine were observed clinically as a part of making diagnoses in the sixteenth century, but not until 1684, when an English physician, Thomas Willis, suggested evaporating, distilling, and precipitating urine, was chemistry thought to enhance the understanding of disease. At about the same time, Willis's contemporary, Robert Boyle, was calling for the chemical analysis of blood. Additionally, in 1722, the serum and solid components of blood were being investigated by William Hewson, an English medical scientist, and interest was developing in the blood chemistry of diabetes.

Richard Bright, an English doctor, forged a critical link between chemistry and anatomy in 1827, when he discovered that "dropsy" patients had damaged kidneys and high albumen levels in their urine [17]. The disease was renamed as Bright's disease, and the fact that there are significant chemical signs of major diseases was established.

Pathological anatomy, at least since Morgagni, had searched for change in the solid parts of the body, drawing attention away from body fluids, partly as a reaction against humoral theories of disease. Hence, Reiser argues, chemical analysis at first was considered to be a special type of dissection, which detected the diseases missed by the pathologist during an autopsy [5, pp. 122-143]. Wanting to avoid being identified with humoral theorists, chemists formed close collegial bonds with microbiologists and the microscope formed their shared instrumental connection.

In 1841, a French physician, Gabriel Andral, described the circumstances that altered the proportions of the blood's components in anemia, plethora, diabetes, and gout. Identifying the chemical components of urine were proceeding in parallel studies by other chemists. Counting red cells in the blood was introduced in 1850, and counting red corpuscles as a method of predicting anemia was established in 1877. The value of chemical tests in diagnosis increased during the 1880s and 1890s, and the collaboration of bacteriology and chemistry paid off in the chemical detection of typhoid fever [18, pp. 363-373]. The white cell became an object of intensive study during this period, thus generating an early scientific understanding of the body's immune system. And in 1901, a successful test for syphilis was discovered.

The establishment of clinical laboratories at the end of the nineteenth century brought biological and physical scientists directly into medicine. The first clinical chemical laboratories in the United States were at Ann Arbor, Michigan (1893) and Philadelphia (1895). Laboratories appeared eventually in hospital wards, government public health organizations, and private businesses related to health care. Reiser points out that "delegating medical decisions to laboratory specialists . . . added certainty to the diagnosis of many diseases" [5, p. 143]. However, his point is that the role of basic science in diagnosis had grown to the point that the physician's self-confidence in making independent diagnostic decisions was beginning to be undermined. Science was producing such specialized data that no primary care physician could understand all of this information. Clinical judgments came to be mistrusted, unless they were accompanied by extremely technical information. This growth of scientific medicine in the nineteenth century, therefore, led to the proliferation of specialties witnessed during the twentieth.

IMPLICATIONS OF THE GROWTH OF SCIENCE AND TECHNOLOGY

The accomplishments of scientific medicine in the second half of the nineteenth century were remarkable. In the 1880s, the organisms responsible for key epidemics (tuberculosis, cholera, typhoid fever, and diphtheria) were isolated. Microbiology allowed physicians to establish the links between disease and cause, between diagnosis and treatment. So completely were these connections imprinted on the popular mind that germ theory, and the specific etiology perspective of the biomedical model, came to dominate scientific medicine and raise hopes that disease would soon be eradicated from the earth, or at least from the civilized world. By the 1890s, clinical medicine was actually making a difference in people's health, although these improvements resulted primarily from prevention and other advancements in public health [19].

Most persons do not realize that the Johns Hopkins School of Medicine opened its doors only a century ago in 1893. This school was the first of its kind and still serves as a prototype for medical schools. Hopkins offered a medical program that constituted a graduate education in basic science and hospital medicine, with equal time spent in labs and on wards. Additionally, advanced residences were offered in specialized fields. This development took place at a time when most medical schools drew their faculty from local physicians, and required little for admission beyond a high school degree and the ability to pay. But this was also a time when states were codifying and escalating the educational component of their licensing requirements. Great optimism was also present about achieving the goals of scientific medicine, especially with regard to finding cures for acute infectious diseases.

Paul Starr contends that in 1904 the American Medical Association's newly established Council on Medical Education sought to close the many small proprietary medical schools, and to encourage, in their place, the development of schools based on the Johns Hopkins model [5, pp. 112-123]. The Council began rating graduate schools according to the scores their graduates achieved on licensing exams. This rating process forced some schools into bankruptcy, and change was slow. The Carnegie Foundation sent Abraham Flexner, a young educational reformer, to site visit each of the nation's medical schools, accompanied by the secretary of the AMA Council on Medical Education, and make recommendations based on what he found.

By the time Flexner wrote his famous *Bulletin Number Four* in 1910, scientific medicine had become the primary mode of investigating and treating disease. Starr calculates that "at most, Flexner hastened the schools to their graves and deprived them of mourners" [5, p. 120]. Consolidation was already proceeding. He argued, agreeing with the AMA, that all medical schools should be closed except those training the scientist-physician [20]. Indeed, he would have reduced the 131 schools to thirty-one. Nonetheless, over twice that number survived. This reorganization of medical education had implications beyond the training of physicians. The entire edifice of professional medicine took shape. These changes were consistent with the rise of positivism and the belief in the ability of this methodology to procure objectively valid knowledge. As a result of Flexner, the emphasis was on adapting medicine to the most advanced intervention technology, and rejecting those approaches that did not champion the use of these devices [21]. Furthermore, Rockefeller's General Educational board, through its philanthropic efforts, sought to impose a model of medical education that was more closely wedded to research than to clinical practice. In fact, most doctors trained after 1920 have a hard time distinguishing between science and medicine.

To be sure, medicine's total embrace of science has had profound positive effects, but the growth of scientific medicine also has a significant down side due to an overdependence on technology. Laboratory analyses in the second half of the twentieth century have become increasingly automated. A classic example is the use of the x-ray. With the introduction of computers into x-ray tomography, and the invention of magnetic resonance imaging, physicians can locate disease in the body with greater clarity and ease than was possible earlier. One difficulty with the continuous advance of diagnostic technology is the correspondingly escalating reliance on technical tools, thus bringing about the atrophy of actual clinical skills. Doctors may actually be deskilled by the rise of high-tech instruments. Accordingly, during the 1920s there was already a concern about excessive diagnostic inquisitiveness. By the 1950s, the term "shot-gun testing" was used. As the century progressed, more was heard about defensive medicine being practiced to protect physicians from potential malpractice suits. To a certain extent, the patient-physician relationship has come to be dictated by technical advances [5, pp. 158-173].

Faith in science and technology is strong in clinical medicine. Doctors see themselves as using the same rigorous methods as scientists. Recording medical facts quantitatively in charts and graphs seems very exact and final. In point of fact, physicians sound like scientists when they describe symptoms or functions in quantitative, rather than qualitative, terms.

This underlying faith in science, again, is the dark side of medicine. The proliferation of technology and scientific medicine, the reduction of answers to cells, then to molecular levels, and the increasing reliance on the opinions of specialists have all tended to make diagnoses abstract. Reiser contends that the impersonality of the physician-patient relationship, and the wall of technology that the physician stands behind, may be like ego defenses, or ways of shielding medical personnel from facing their own limitations as healers [5, pp. 227-231]. When a diagnosis boils down to choosing which tests to order and which specialists to consult, what happens to the skill level of physicians? Doctors can easily become masters of technique and insensitive to the patient's "soul," as Frankl notes [22]. They may become divorced systematically from the social context of medicine. And no matter how many attempts are made to remove medicine from cultural exigencies, health and illness remain existential issues. What could be more personal than the concern for one's well-being?

Scientific medicine since the 1930s has been more interested in the biochemistry of disease than in undertaking real comprehensive physical examinations, as reflected in medical school curricula. Nowadays both physical examinations and medical history taking are being delegated increasingly to nurse practitioners and physician's assistants, as group practice allows real science to be left to doctors. Specialization has thus expanded to the extent that physicians have become merely intermediaries between patients, technicians, and machines. Physicians have become functionaries in an increasingly arcane system [23].

In a certain sense, the biomedical model carries within itself the seeds of its demise. As the twentieth century dawned, the model had much success. Due to its accomplishments in the realm of infectious diseases, biomedicine had a lot of support. During the second half of the twentieth century, however, the biomedical model became strained. The dualism, materialism, and reductionism, for example, that brought about progress in medicine were called into question. These qualities were anathema to the holism desired by the public.

But the crisis witnessed during the 1960s, 1970s, and 1980s may pale by comparison to the trend that looms on the horizon. As the U.S. population ages, the limited scope of biomedicine will experience unprecedented strain. The chronic illnesses of older persons, simply put, will require a shift away from the limitations of the biomedical model, if medical intervention is to be efficacious. In other words, the traits that made biomedicine so effective in the nineteenth century and early in the twentieth, impede intervention with chronic disease. This story is told in the following chapter.

REFERENCES

1. R. M. Zaner, *Ethics and the Clinical Encounter,* Prentice Hall, Englewood Cliffs, New Jersey, 1988.
2. M. Foucault, *The Birth of the Clinic,* Pantheon, New York, 1973.
3. L. J. Rather, Toward a Philosophical Study of the Idea of Disease, in *The Historical Development of Physiological Thought,* C. M. Brooks and P. F. Cranefield (eds.), Macmillan (Hafner Press) New York, pp. 351-373, 1959.
4. H. E. Sigerist, *Medicine and Human Welfare,* Yale University Press, New Haven, 1945.
5. S. J. Reiser, *Medicine and the Reign of Technology,* Cambridge University Press, London, 1978.

6. W. R. Arney and B. J. Bergen, *Medicine and the Management of Living,* University of Chicago Press, Chicago, 1984.
7. E. J. Cassell, *The Nature of Suffering and the Goals of Medicine,* Oxford University Press, New York, 1991.
8. G. B. Morgagni, *The Seats and Causes of Diseases Investigated by Anatomy,* B. Alexander (trans.) 1769, Macmillan (Hafner Press), New York, 1960.
9. S. Lehrer, *Explorers of the Body,* Doubleday, Garden City, New York, 1979.
10. P. Starr, *The Social Transformation of American Medicine,* Basic Books, New York, 1982.
11. S. B. Nuland, *Doctors,* Knopf, New York, 1988.
12. S. J. Reiser, Technologic Environments as Causes of Suffering: The Ethical Context, in *The Hidden Dimension of Illness: Human Suffering,* P. L. Starck and J. P. McGovern (eds.), National League for Nursing Press, New York, 1992.
13. R. Barthes, *Camera Lucida,* Hill and Wang, New York, 1981.
14. C. Herzlich and J. Pierret, *Illness and Self in Society,* The Johns Hopkins University Press, Baltimore, 1987.
15. I. Galdston, *Progress in Medicine,* Knopf, New York, pp. 46-84, 1940.
16. P. De Kruif, *Microbe Hunters,* Harcourt Brace and Co., New York, 1926.
17. B. J. Ficarra, *Essays on Historical Medicine,* Froben Press, New York, pp. 158-159, 1948.
18. L. Clendening, *Behind the Doctor,* The Garden City Publishing Co., Garden City, New York, 1933.
19. R. Dubos, *Mirage of Health,* Harper and Row, New York, pp. 95-128, 1959.
20. A. Flexner, *Medical Education in the United States and Canada,* Bulletin No. 4. Carnegie Foundation for the Advancement of Teaching, New York, 1910.
21. M. Kaufman, Homeopathy in America: The Rise and Fall and Persistence of a Medical Herecy, in *Other Healers,* N. Gevitz (ed.), The Johns Hopkins University Press, Baltimore, pp. 99-123, 1988.
22. V. Frankl, *Doctor of the Soul,* Alfred A. Knopf, New York, 1963.
23. A. R. Jonsen, *The New Medicine and the Old Ethics,* Harvard University Press, Cambridge, Massachusetts, pp. 24ff, 1990.

CHAPTER
5

Aging and Paradigm Strain

In his analysis of American health policy, Fox describes an imaginary scene in 1895 in which prominent physicians and leading philanthropists gather for the purpose of setting priorities for policy in the next century. Agreement is quickly reached that the major focus of health policy should be "preventing and alleviating the pain and poverty caused by acute infectious diseases and two chronic infections, tuberculosis and syphilis" [1, p. 3]. Everyone in the room could remember the discoveries of Robert Koch and Louis Pasteur. The other diseases that should be conquered were diphtheria, typhoid fever, typhus, and pneumonia. In this regard, they easily agreed that health policy should prioritize research in the areas of bacteriology, physiology, and related sciences.

Another important issue is related to renovating and building general acute care hospitals. These would be places where the latest scientific findings and the newest medical technology, including the recently invented x-ray machine, could be applied to the diagnosis and treatment of patients. Medical schools should also be reformed, so that they could engage in medical research as well as teach laboratory science, supervise clinical training on the wards, and prepare clinicians in scientific medicine for the future century. As mentioned in the previous chapter, Johns Hopkins and Harvard would be the model. In sum, health policy at the turn of the century was designed to increase the supply of useful scientific knowledge, appropriate facilities, and trained personnel for acute care. This orientation represented a triumph in health policy, and testified to the stunningly successful biomedical model.

The health policy put in place at the turn of the twentieth century worked well. Medical research and education expanded, thereby increasing the supply of scientifically trained physicians who would value and use the newest biomedical technology and related approaches. The number of hospitals, housing diagnostic and treatment equipment, grew rapidly throughout the century, as did this technology. As a result, acute infectious diseases were no longer the leading killers by the 1920s.[1] Science had triumphed. But by 1940, another trend was firmly in place. Acute diseases were replaced as leading the causes of death by the same chronic diseases that lead the list today: heart disease, cancer, and stroke.[2]

THE SHIFT FROM ACUTE TO CHRONIC DISEASE

The challenges of today are different than they were a century ago. Most acute infections have been conquered, along with key chronic diseases such as tuberculosis and syphilis. Nonetheless, there is no simple inoculation for the major killers today (heart disease, stroke, and cancer). These problems may be prevented and managed, but they have defied cure.

But despite radical changes in the disease landscape, the priorities of 1900 remain in place today. Stated simply, the health care system in the United States is still focused primarily on acute care. Even in the case of the major killing diseases, for example, little formal attention and resources are given to their prevention. And only a minority of all physicians in the United States today focus on primary care and give much attention to disease management. Indeed, according to the biomedical model, interventions that are not aimed at cure are considered suspect.

The health care system has grown in complexity during the twentieth century, thus generating many professional and business interests. So when Fox imagined a meeting today to consider the health policy of the next century, he imagined an auditorium, not a board

[1] The Committee on Public Health of the New York Academy of Medicine reported in 1914 that more people were dying of chronic illnesses than acute, as quoted in Fox [1, p. 32].

[2] The rise of heart disease, cancer, and stroke to the top of the list of killer diseases by 1940 was reported by Fox, and derived from *Vital Statistics in the United States, 1940-1960*, Washington DC: Department of Health, Education and Welfare, National Center for Health Statistics, 1968) [1, p. 79].

room, in which sat not only physicians (primarily leaders of dozens of professional specialty groups) and philanthropists (foundation directors), but also many entrepreneurs and special interests who would not have been present a century earlier. These would include representatives of professional nursing and basic medical science associations. Additionally, business managers of large hospitals, hospital chains, health maintenance organizations, nursing homes and home health care agencies would be there, as well as representatives of pharmaceutical, medical supply, and equipment companies (and trade associations created by these groups). Economists and ethicists, government representatives from the state and federal levels, and representatives of nonprofit and commercial insurance companies, public interest organizations, unions, and many lawyers and journalists would also be vying for attention. Indeed, only a minority of persons in the room would be physicians. All of these groups would be less interested in achieving a new consensus on health policy than in achieving and protecting their respective interests in the health care system.

The medical landscape has changed. The biomedical empire designed in the last century has been built, but the social environment has dramatically changed. Chronic disease is on the rise, while acute problems, except for AIDS, seem to require less attention. With people living longer, this trend will only continue. This shift has created considerable pressure on biomedicine, due to internal paradigm strain and external pressure from patients, business, and government. Change will have to occur, or the medical enterprise may become even more burdensome or, possibly, less relevant.

PRESSURES FROM THE INSIDE: IS OBJECTIVITY ILLUSORY?

What gives the current health policy such incredible staying power, despite its increasing cost and decreasing returns? In addition to all of the economic interests that turn the flywheel of American health policy, there are epistemological forces that also keep the medical system in place. The classic science worldview on which biomedicine rests has changed relatively little over the century. Further, science has a vocabulary that ignores the everyday world. This language is about disease, whose causes are physical, located in the human body, and require interventions that target a person's physiology. Specifically noteworthy, this language was initially designed by biomedical scientists to deal with curative medicine. Unfortunately, this *modus operandi* does not yield easily to other understandings of the patient, disease etiology, or treatment.

Science is not always objective, straightforward, or compelling, despite what the general public is told. Even within the realm of science, doubts abound. The objectivity of measures secured from biomedical technology, for example, is assumed in most interventions. To be sure, the ability to provide standardized data on biological functions and biochemistry was a big step forward in the nineteenth century. Reliable information was thus made available on a large scale. During the twentieth century, however, the naive trust in the objectivity of physical data has been challenged. There is a greater awareness now that all observations have a subjective component. They are recorded and interpreted by humans, even if this input is collected and displayed by machines. Observer error and technical errors are always likely to be present. And interpretation varies depending on the physician's medical education, experience, and knowledge about the techniques that are used.

For example, Reiser reports several discouraging studies on accuracy. The Center for Disease Control, in the mid-1960s, put laboratory accuracy at about 25 percent [2]. Currently, laboratory accuracy remains a widely debated issue, despite equipment automation. One study, conducted during World War II, found that physicians disagreed with one another's reading of x-rays about one-third of the time [3 (cited in 2, p. 190)], and in a 1958 study agreement on EKG tracings was about the same [4 (cited in 2, p. 190)]. In 1960, heart specialists were able to identify heart abnormalities correctly only 79 percent of the time using stethoscopes; primary care physicians did worse [5 (cited in 2, p. 191)].

The same issues are present in medicine today. In a special issue of *Communications in Statistics: Theory and Methods,* devoted to drug testing, Follmann, Wu, and Geller argue that variations and instrumental configurations can cause the findings of highly sophisticated drug testing equipment to be misinterpreted, yielding false positives and false negatives [6]. Knowledge of the advantages and pitfalls of different types of testing systems is necessary in order to avoid mistakes. Most clinicians, of course, lack this knowledge. When an average batch of urine samples are tested repeatedly on the same machines, there is only 93 to 95 percent agreement [7]. When assessing symptoms, apparently physicians often see what they expect to find. But subsequent to the discovery of the uncertainty principle in quantum theory by Heisenberg, and other modern developments in epistemology, this self-fulfilling prophesy is not surprising [8]. Initial assumptions, in short, play a large role in the collection of data and reporting of findings. Reality depends on one's starting point.

PRESSURE FROM THE INSIDE: NAGGING DOUBTS ABOUT THE SINGLE FOCUS ON THE BODY

But more fundamental problems have begun to plague scientists. There is also an uneasiness in medicine about the true efficacy of the biomedical model, a point discussed by Foss and Rothenberg [9]. Physicians understand that real cures come more rarely and dearly today, and that chronic disease, at best, can be prevented or postponed. Also understood is that after their onset, such diseases must be managed. Accordingly, distinctions are made in medical schools between preventive and curative, chronic and acute diseases and conditions for and causes of disease.[3] Given these distinctions, physicians have begun to admit that a cure may be impossible in many instances. And with the rise in chronic conditions, cures may become rarer.

Advocates of biomedicine were shocked when one third of Americans were rejected from military service in World War II for emotional and psychological disorders [10 (summarized in 2, pp. 179-180)]. Since that time, psychiatrists and medical social workers have reminded physicians of the fact that patients are biopsychosocial beings, and not just bodies. Nowadays, because of the findings of behavioral medicine [11], there is a grudging awareness that patients can react physiologically to stress. Physicians are also aware of the behavioral and lifestyle risk factors of disease; in this regard, epidemiologists have begun to question the limitations of biomedicine. As Freund and McGuire relate, "With its broad generalizations, social epidemiology sets the stage for a more refined analysis of the ways a society produces, defines, experiences, and treats sickness and death" [12, p. 35]. Practitioners have begun to acknowledge, in a variety of instances, that disease relates to

---

[3] In their chapter on responses to the limitations of biomedicine, Foss and Rothenberg argue that adopting the tenets of the biomedical model has not blinded physicians to the existence of other ways of looking at disease, and that many of them realize the limitations of this model. Their point is that physicians are trapped in the biomedical model, and are unable to break loose from it because there is no viable paradigm that works as well to define the parameters of science.

a host of factors, which are minimally related to physiology. In some quarters, at least, the old dualism has already begun to break down.

Nonetheless, as Foss and Rothenberg point out, extrasomatic considerations cannot be examined using the formal vocabulary of science [9, pp. 114-132]. And although the multi-causal basis of disease is widely recognized, medical research is routinely limited to studying biophysical causes. But at practically every turn anomalies arise. Persons change their diets and get better; an environmental change affects positively an individual's health; and will power holds a disease at bay. How persons define themselves alters their activity level, outlook, and susceptibility to disease [13].

PRESSURE FROM THE OUTSIDE:
MEDICAL COUNTERMOVEMENTS

Despite this evidence, the orthodoxy of the biomedical model remains, for the most part, a fortress. Because of the limitations and exclusiveness of orthodox biomedicine, three other approaches to health and illness have arisen outside the fortress's walls. Foss and Rothenberg describe them as medical countermovements that try to extend biomedicine's narrow focus [9, pp. 83-88]. They are holistic, environmental, and behavioral medicine. Each of the three countermovements is understood to be reacting to the limitations of the biomedical model, but not as splinter groups. Instead, they are gaining widespread acceptance among the public. Furthermore, their adherents publish in journals, often have M.D.'s or Ph.D.'s, and conduct research funded by federal agencies.

Of the three, holistic medicine is the least accepted by practitioners of orthodox biomedicine, because this more encompassing approach is more concerned with the sick person than the diseased body. Proponents of holism complain that biomedicine focuses too much on the somatic nature of disease, rather than viewing patients as spiritual, psychological and cultural, as well as physical beings, who relate dynamically to their social and physical environments. Holistic medicine emphasizes "wellness" [14, p. 9]. Information on this perspective is found in the book section of health food stores, as well as elsewhere. Within this framework patients are encouraged to become actively involved in their healing process, rather than being passive recipients of the healer's ministrations. A variety of treatment modalities are accepted that would not be considered reliable by the standards of biomedicine. In general, an ecumenical, inclusive attitude is adopted toward healers. Health maintenance is stressed rather than crisis intervention, including diet, exercise, stress management, and environmental safeguards.

Environmental medicine stands closer to biomedicine than does holistic medicine. According to this option, the causes of disease are understood to emanate from the physical and social environment and afflict or burden the body [9, pp. 114-132]. More concerned with the origin of disease than its "mechanisms," advocates of environmental medicine focus on why a disease occurs. Therefore, they emphasize the environmental, behavioral, and nutritional ways of avoiding disease in the first place. The theoretical base of this approach is rooted in an historical understanding of human evolution and environmental adjustments. That is, individual human biology is less importance than the biology of human populations. Again, from this perspective, the body in isolation is an inappropriate subject of study. Supporters of environmental medicine stress preventive strategies, and are quick to point out that in the nineteenth century, before the discoveries of Koch and Pasteur, the incidence of infectious diseases declined in Europe because of environmental corrections [15]. This view is especially interesting because the biomedical model is assailed on its own turf, i.e., curative medicine. By the way, public health is rooted in environmental medicine.

Of the three countermovements, behavioral medicine stands the closest to biomedicine. Neuroendocrinology and psychoneuroimmunology, for examples, are outgrowths of this approach to medicine. The most basic assumption of this movement, according to Foss and Rothenberg, is that "there is an interrelationship among the immune system, the central nervous system, and the endocrine system" [9, p. 86]. Therefore, mind and body are viewed as two ends of a continuum, and attempts are made to identify neurochemical mechanisms that operate in conjunction with subjective states to trigger physiological reactions.[4] Mind-body dualism is criticized, while multidisciplinary approaches are sought for integrating biological and psychological knowledge. Nonetheless, the mind and the brain are treated as identical, and the mind-body link is often interpreted by the biomedical

---

[4] Behavioral medicine has one foot in biomedicine and the other in holistic medicine. The behavioral framework does not include all of the healing modalities like holistic medicine, and talks the language of biomedicine. The mind-body connection, however, is recognized, along with the efficacy of coping mechanisms to reduce stress. Clearly, biomedicine rejects this approach. So behavioral medicine is truly marginal; sometimes this branch of medicine is included in the fold and sometimes it is rejected.

audience as body(brain)-body interaction. Still, behavioral medicine has contributed greatly to stress research and to understanding the biopsychological connections between stress, personality, coping styles, the immune system and disease. As with holistic and environmental medicine, humans are understood to affect and to be influenced by their social and physical environments.

Attempts have been made to incorporate behavioral medicine into the biomedical model; their meeting place is in psychoneuroimmunology. The way hormones are affected by emotions, and the action of hormones on the immune system, has been demonstrated scientifically to biomedicine's satisfaction. But this association is conceptualized in mechanistic—mostly biochemical—terms that physicians find reasonable [16, p. 55]. On the other hand, treatment strategies that involve the exercise of psychological coping mechanisms to protect the individual from the effect of stressors is beyond the scope of the biomedical model and the language of biomedicine. A volitional element is presupposed by these kinds of interventions that does not conform to a naturalistic view of the mind or body.

PRESSURE FROM THE OUTSIDE:
MEDICAL DEPERSONALIZATION AND CONSUMERISM

Criticism of science became increasingly prevalent during the 1960s and early 1970s, when authority of all kinds was being challenged by a baby boom generation come of age. Medical authority did not escape this onslaught. Physicians seemed less like gods, and their sovereign profession came under fire as epitomizing greed. The escalating cost of medicine and dwindling access to services underscored a public sense of betrayal by both science and professional medicine. Many persons began to believe that scientific medicine was a monopoly designed to keep prices high and avoid competition. In this conspiratorial view, as a result of a great public relations effort, medical knowledge was controlled and kept within a limited circle of experts. Information about treatment, accordingly, became quite esoteric. But this is an exaggerated version of what actually happened, according to some social historians who assign the primary conspirator role to the American Medical Association [17].

Nonetheless, with their narrow focus on the body and over-dependence on medical technology, doctors had become more and more removed from a real relationship with the patients. The importance of taking in-depth medical histories and talking with patients about their illness experience declined, as a by-product of the praise lavished on technical developments. Accordingly, the quality of the interaction between patients and physicians began to be impersonal and strained. But when doctor-patient relationships are not personally satisfying, because the doctor, as a person, is not relating to the patient as a person, patients are less positive about their treatment and unwilling to comply with the regimen prescribed.[5] And because scientific detachment was no longer offset by unquestioning trust in the scientist-physician, malpractice suits increased. Patients, simply put, began to feel misunderstood, isolated, and manipulated. In fact, Zaner argues that the growing distance between doctors and patients in the twentieth century is traceable directly to the influence of the biomedical model [18].

This issue is critically important in the context of chronic illness. Doctors may give lower priority to managing patients' chronic conditions because this mode of treatment requires that they spend a lot of time talking with patients, and engaging in a significant amount of work that is ostensibly non-scientific. According to Fox, however, doctors should have a lot to talk about [1]. They should advise about preventing or postponing disease; take detailed medical histories that facilitate making early diagnoses; assist in behavioral modification; educate patients about treatment regimens; and discuss options that could reduce disability, e.g., among drugs, devices, and modifications of home and workplace.[6] Because of the distance required between the

---

[5] This point is made excellently by Eric Cassell in a chapter on the clinical experience in *The Nature of Suffering and the Goals of Medicine,* Oxford Press, London, 1991. He argues that it is not just medical knowledge that is important, but the experience of the physician as a person, and the ability to relate to the patient as a person, that is the key to successful clinical practice. Arthur Kleinman, Leon Eisenberg and Byron Good, "Culture, Illness and Care," *Annals of Internal Medicine, 88,* 1978, make a similar point in distinguishing between disease and illness. Furthermore, patients cooperate better with doctors when the doctor responds to their illness experience, not just to their disease. The authors of this book have heard long-practiced clinicians in internal medicine remark that malpractice suits and stubborn noncompliance indicate a failure to relate to the patient as a person. Cassell would call this the "art" rather than the "science" of medicine; he sees the two as often in conflict, which is the position held also by the authors of this book.

[6] These activities take too much time, in the view of most physicians. Cynics sometimes assert that talking to patients holds down the doctor's income, because more patients can be seen when discussion time is reduced. If a physician's assistant or nurse practitioner works in the practice, they will be delegated nearly all of these tasks. And when these "physician extenders" are not present, many jobs will be delegated to nurses. Fox argues that these are tasks that physicians should value, particularly when dealing with patients who suffer from chronic diseases in their pre-clinical stages.

caregiver and patient by the biomedical model, most specialists and many primary care physicians find this kind of activity difficult to justify [19, 20]. In the end, however, patients are denied the intimacy they desire with their physicians.

Furthermore, during the Reagan administration there was a tendency to recognize medicine as an industry and encourage market mechanisms to control costs. Physicians were called "providers" and hospitals "provider organizations." Consistent with this outlook, patients were called "health care consumers." Corporate medicine created the circumstances and the consumer protection movement the values that inundated health care during the 1980s. Together they provided a setting in which the doctor-patient relationship came to be seen as commercial, impersonal, and contractual. But clearly the values and attitudes that subtend commercial relationships are pragmatic and self-interested, and not idealistic. This shift eroded further the authority of the physician.

Fox, in tracing health policy in this century, contends that medicine had always had a special relationship with business. Wealthy businessmen formed the philanthropies that encouraged the institutional development of scientific medicine in the United States. Additionally, they offered medical insurance to their employees, thereby increasing the employees' loyalty to, and dependence on, the employer. The government blessed this special relationship by not taxing medical benefits. Fox notes that this special relationship began to deteriorate in the late 1970s and 1980s, when American businesses became anxious about the state of the economy [1, pp. 94-101]. The cost of health care increased, while profits diminished. Accordingly, employers began treating health care exactly as they would any other commodity by self-insuring under provisions of the 1974 Employee Retirement and Income Security Act, and negotiating discounts for their employees from physicians and hospitals.

This maneuvering conveyed to the public the idea that health care was not something personal, but merely a commodity. Health care, simply put, is not integrated into daily life, but is something that is periodically consumed. Rather than maintained, health is purchased from employers and the doctors they retain.

Along with this commodification of health care, a sort of symbolic association began to develop between businesses and medicine. Certain joint ventures by physicians, for example, became a common place. Fox reports that a 1992 study in Florida found that ". . . 40 percent of the physicians in direct patient care had an investment interest in a health care business to which they may refer their patients for services" [21 (cited in 1, p. 99)]. Employees, in the meanwhile, were increasingly regarding health care as a con game, thereby further diminishing the moral stature of the medical profession. The health of persons seemed to many to be in the hands of callous profiteers, and thus patients tried to take advantage of the medical system at every opportunity. As might be expected, fraud became a regular part of providing care.

The consumer protection movement of the 1970s is credited with generating the political pressure to diminish the power of physicians and increase the stature of the patient in the doctor-patient relationship. What had seemed as "beneficence" by physicians came increasingly to be viewed as "paternalism."

In a related issue, reports of the abuse of power by medical researchers gave rise to the 1973 National Commission on the Protection of Human Subjects, according to Rothman [22, pp. 85-100]. This commission sought to eliminate studies where subjects were studied without their knowledge, sometimes in ways that damaged their health. This board revolutionized human research by requiring researchers to get permission from subjects before including them in studies. The 1978 President's Commission for the Study of Ethical Problems in Medicine and Biomedical and Behavioral Research, the successor organization to the human subjects commission, grappled with the ethics of decision-making in the context of medical treatment. A key conclusion was that such decision-making must be shared between the doctor and the patient, but in the end the patient has the final word on a course of action. In the 1983 report entitled *Deciding to Forego Life-sustaining Treatment,* the point was made that hospitals should formulate "explicit, and publicly available policies regarding how and by whom decisions are made" [23, p. 205].[7] At least where there is a clash of wills between physicians and their patients today, the law is on the patient's side. The consumer movement, therefore, blunted the one doctrine of the biomedical model that states that the body is the proper location of regimen and control and that the physician applies the control. In fact, Fox believes that Americans may already be questioning, *en masse,* the authority of physicians, as evidenced by patients "limiting their consumption of useless and expensive services at the end of their lives . . . [1, p. 118]. And most recently, the passage of the American with Disabilities Act in 1990 may force the

---

[7] This report is discussed and quoted in [22, pp. 85-100].

health care establishment to deal with patients in a more responsible and humane way.

The point must be made at this juncture, however, that these changes are occurring at the periphery of medicine. If care is ever going to be significantly expanded, critical reflection on the core of traditional medicine will have to be inaugurated. Accordingly, alternatives to biomedicine will not be inferiorized simply because they do not fall within the parameters established by science.

Biomedicine is currently more vulnerable to change than ever before. Nonetheless, alternatives will not be given a fair hearing until the basic philosophy and entire array of traditional medical practices are open to review. Everything must be put on the table, so to speak, before real medical reform will occur.

PRESSURE FROM THE OUTSIDE: THE OLD AGE CHALLENGE

In 1994, major health care reform seems to be on the horizon in the United States. This movement is likely to alter access to health care in a major way, and perhaps hold costs to a manageable growth rate in the future. A greater change in biomedicine, however, is likely to occur in the second decade of the next century when the older population of the United States grows enormously, because of the aging of the baby boom generation that was born between 1946 and 1964. The crisis precipitated by this eventuality may be large enough to create a paradigm shift away from the biomedical model. In this way, physicians may be forced to temper their enthusiasm for biomedicine, despite their usual resistance to change.

The growth of the older population is relevant to biomedicine, because chronic illnesses tend to accumulate with advancing old age. Epidemiologist Maurice Mittelmark made this point clearly when he asserted that

> accident and injury are prominent concerns in childhood, adolescence and early adulthood, developing chronic diseases are a central feature of middle adulthood, morbidity and mortality from chronic diseases characterize the period around retirement, and deterioration in functioning, disability and dependency are concerns mainly of old and very old age [24, pp. 135-151].

Functional ability tends to decline eventually for very old persons as impairment leads to disability and disability leads to handicap status, thereby requiring increasingly comprehensive levels of care that make treatment in advanced old age potentially an expensive proposition. Age magnifies need not only for the aging persons, but for their care-givers and for society as a whole. Most important, however, is the kind of need that is increased in populations, if not necessarily in persons, by aging.

Unfortunately, this is not the sort of condition that biomedicine is designed to meet. What is required is chronic, not acute, care. For example, preventive strategies are called for to delay and diminish health crises, while rehabilitation and disease management strategies are needed afterwards. Environmental and holistic approaches stand ready to step into the breech, but these are exactly the areas of medi-cine that challenge the limitations of the biomedical model.

The biomedical model, along with the most recent attempt to com-modify medicine, work in tandem to deal ineffectively with chronic disease. With the emphasis placed on cure, along with medical research focusing on the search for magic bullets, patients are treated ineffec-tively and cost continues to rise. More effective and less costly interven-tions are available, but their use, at least initially, does not appear to be medically or economically sound.

Long-term care is the phrase that is used to capture the image of functional maintenance for the aging population.[8] The rapid growth of the older population will carry a similar acceleration of the long-term care population, and will challenge the biomedical model in a very major way. Even long-term care has been defined by the language of biomedicine, as "institutional and noninstitutional services for people with chronic conditions that are marked by a pronounced deviation from a normal state of health and are manifested in discomforting, abnormal physical or mental conditions" [25]. In other words, chronic disease is defined as a departure from normal physiological function-ing, from which substantial recovery is possible in the long run. None-theless, the current approach of battling heroically to save lives after the consequences of chronic disease have reached a crisis stage, and,

---

[8] The long-term care concept is the primary focus of health services for the elderly; this idea includes the full range of care, including preventive care, supportive services, treatment, rehabilitation, and several levels of nursing care. This is a comprehensive term, and as such is difficult for biomedicine to handle. For example, supportive services, unless they are explicitly medical, would not be considered as health care. The key to understanding long-term care is the concept of functional ability. As functional ability declines, various levels of support and care are needed to offset this reduction, and restore as much functioning as is possible.

ignoring all else, will be challenged by the demand that is coming in the future.

Long-term care is often conceptualized as a continuum that ranges downward from skilled nursing care at a nursing home, to informal assistance provided by family and friends from the community, with formal medical and supportive services supplied in the home lying somewhere in between these options [26]. Relatively little of this care, under present biomedical definitions, would be considered "strictly medical." Specifically, this broader range of services strive to "achieve harmony on social and personal levels," which mainstream physicians are loathe to recognize as medical [27, p. 20]. These practices are treated by many physicians as merely social or cultural accoutrements, which serve to supplement standard medical interventions.

There have been many studies that attempt to define the size and characteristics of the prevailing long-term care population, primarily through surveys of various kinds. These efforts are prompted by the interest of government in controlling costs, by the concerns of planners and policy makers for identifying future needs and costs, and by the practice community in providing an appropriate level of care to functionally disabled elders. These strategies, however, are usually motivated by medical concerns. The result has been that the actual needs and experiences of citizens are masked or misconstrued. The proliferation of services aimed at acute care, that do not make sense, has become the norm.

Biomedicine, because so little is invested in the prevention and management of chronic disease in the community, tends to push older persons into higher levels of medical care than they actually need. Studies have shown that from 20 to 40 percent of those in nursing homes could be served as effectively by appropriate community-based services or in a nursing home at a lower level of intensity [28, 29]. In fact, elders prefer overwhelmingly to remain at home when possible, where they can maintain a greater sense of interdependence with family members, friends, and neighbors, and a lesser sense of dependency [30, 31]. Others estimate that 800,000 to 1,400,000 persons over age sixty-five need long-term care in some form but are not receiving this kind of service [32].

Because of the limitations of the biomedical model, and the control of health care by the medical profession, medicare reimburses for only a limited range of skilled nursing and rehabilitation services, though studies indicate a larger need for personal care and household management services [33]. Need for care in one's home increases with age and is related to a progressive loss of functional ability. But note should be taken that the relationship between disability and need for home care varies according to the type and severity of the disability, as well as on the age, adaptability, and resources of the individual in question. A strict medical rule of thumb, in short, has not worked when trying to estimate the appropriateness of home care.

According to the National Center for Health Statistics, some 12 percent of all the community-dwelling persons over sixty-five require some form of home health care services. Of all the persons who need home care services, about one-third have celebrated their seventy-fifth birthday [34, 35]. Furthermore, Kart and Dunkle report that most elderly persons who live at home assess their own capacity to provide self-care to be high. Only 11 percent give a fair or poor assessment of their capacity to take care of themselves, which is about the same proportion found to need home care services by the National Center for Health Statistics [36].

Epidemiologists have illustrated that members of certain populations are "at risk" of later entering a diseased state or becoming more disabled by existing diseases.[9] But these nuances of disease are obscured by biomedicine. The biomedical model tends to dichotomize disease and non-disease, and to see the purpose of medicine as diagnosing and treating disease through appropriate physical interventions. But the identification of disease is not this clear-cut, particularly in the case of pre-clinical chronic conditions. Concerning chronic disease, each person is constantly at risk; the *degree* of risk is the critical variable. But the exploration of these risk factors, and ways of eliminating or reducing them, is deemphasized if not rejected by biomedicine. These variables are fuzzy, not easily classified, and difficult to attack with the sureness that one attacks the final, full-blown disease state. Environmental medicine, however, is very interested in just

---

[9] Here epidemiology and environmental medicine blend together in their search for the underlying causes of disease. Epidemiologists follow procedures similar to Morgagni's pathophysiological approach, discussed in Chapter 4, and discover the cause of death in autopsy then argue backward in time to identify the symptoms or disease that brought about a patient's demise. Epidemiology, however, investigates sick populations and not sick individuals. This diagnostic tool of environmental medicine examines the rates of death from diseases, and then works backward to discover those life conditions that are "associated with" or that statistically predict a disease or death. If populations that smoke have higher death rates from lung cancer, then smoking is a risk factor for lung cancer. The more strongly these factors predict death, the more robust the risk factor.

this issue. Nonetheless, attempts to reduce the burden of chronic illness in a rapidly expanding older population will require the greater legitimation of environmental medicine, along with a shift away from over-reliance on biomedical interventions.

Not all persons of any age need or use formal long-term services. However, people who use these services regularly are concentrated in the oldest part of the population. Given the demographic trend that is underway, the current focus of resources, research, and professional attention almost entirely on acute illness cannot continue without disastrous results. Nonetheless, policy makers and health care officials appear to be proceeding as if the American population is not dramatically changing. Yet ignoring this population aging process demonstrates a level of insensitivity that will lead to a health care crisis in the United States of mammoth proportions in a quarter-century, and one that will continue to build between now and then. Demographic evidence to support this point is readily available.

The Senate Special Committee on Aging, the American Association of Retired Persons, the Federal Council on Aging, and the U.S. Administration on Aging published jointly a demographic profile of the elderly population in 1991, with projections to later decades [37]. Perhaps the most basic indicator of population aging is the increase in the relative proportion of older persons in a society's population. Consider, for example, the proportion of the whole U.S. population in different age categories in each of the decades since 1900, and those projected until 2050, when the baby boom generation will have begun to die off in appreciable numbers. During that fifteen-decade period, the population sixty-five years of age or older will have increased from 4 to 22 percent of the U.S. population, or by a multiple of 5.7 times. The population seventy-five to eighty-four years of age will have increased from 1 to 7.2 percent of the national population, an increase of 7.2 times. And the population eighty-five years of age or older will have increased from .2 to 5.1 percent, or 25.5 times its size in 1990.

Not only will the older population have increased in the United States during this time period, but the older population will have also aged. This is an impressive growth curve.

To understand the aging of the older population, the fact should be remembered that different segments of this population are growing at different rates, and therefore they are shifting in their proportions relative to one another. Another way of examining the changes in the size of the older population during these fifteen decades is to consider the shifting proportion of the older population that is very old and more likely to be suffering from multiple chronic illnesses. Those eighty-five years of age and over were only 4 percent of persons sixty-five years of age and over in 1900. Their proportion will have grown to 13 percent by the year 2000, and to 22 percent by 2050. Between 1990 and 2010, the oldest part of the older population will seem to grow especially rapidly. This apparent growth will occur because of the dip in fertility rates during the Great Depression of the 1930s. Therefore, a smaller cohort will begin entering the retirement years during the 1990s, and this will slow the growth of the older population considerably. During the 1990-2000 decade, the growth of the entire retirement-aged population will slow to half of its usual growth rate. However, this slow-down in entry-level retirees will not make the older population stop aging, and this will make the older part of the population seem to grow more rapidly. This rapid aging of the older population will focus attention much more urgently on long-term care issues than in earlier decades, and this attention may result in the first outlines of a national response to the real long-term care crisis that will occur three decades later when the baby boom generation begins entering the oldest old-age group.

But knowing that the older population is growing and aging is not sufficient to provide this group with appropriate services. In order to provide budgetary support for services to that portion of the population in the greatest need of assistance, long-term care planners must know more about the characteristics of the population over age eighty-five and the changes in these traits over time.

The study of population characteristics offers only a skeletal vision of the future. This is because changes in numbers per se do not translate easily and directly into a forecast of total resources. Only the very naive, for example, would infer an X percent increase in units of long-term care service from an increase in the number of very old persons. Diversity within the older population, both present and future, proves the undoing of such simple logic. Contrary to popular stereotypes, not all of the elderly, not even the oldest part, are socially, physically, or economically dependent. Indeed, aging is characterized by increasing variance among individuals; that is, basic physiological markers show more variance within a "normal" range with increasing age [38-40].

While most elders are not acutely ill, the experience of chronic disease at some time is almost inevitable. Prevention and health maintenance, therefore, will become increasingly more relevant. This method of intervention will offset the effect of the rapid growth of the very old population. But most important for this discussion, this strategy is congenial to environmental medicine, that is, to public health.

What are the most common chronic diseases whose prevalence increases with age in old age? They are coronary heart disease, stroke, hypertension, cancer, and osteoporosis. Each of these will be discussed briefly to provide a context for discussing the importance of prevention and maintenance [24].

Coronary heart disease is the leading cause of death and disability among the elderly. This malady has declined steadily over the past two decades, but still remains high. Epidemiological research, at this point, identifies high systolic blood pressure, a particular lipid profile (cholesterol), smoking, diabetes, and educational level as the most important risk factors associated with this disease [24, pp. 142-145]. Most important to note is that chronic diseases are often interactive. Heart disease, in other words, can be indirectly approached by preventing and controlling hypertension and diabetes.

The frequency of stroke increases with age, although trends in death caused by stroke are high but gradually declining [24, p. 148]. The proportion of persons living after strokes in a disabled condition, however, is increasing. Long-term care needs, particularly those centered on rehabilitation, tend to increase following strokes in old age. Much of the improvement of morbidity and mortality is due to improved control of hypertension, again demonstrating an interactive effect with other chronic diseases.

Hypertension, implicated in both heart disease and stroke, increases with age, particularly systolic hypertension [24, p. 146]. This condition can be managed through medications, but more importantly improvement can be witnessed through lifestyle changes aimed at lowering obesity and stress levels and particularly increasing physical fitness through exercise.

Cancers, all sites combined, increase with age, although this disease moderates somewhat among the oldest age group, those over eight-five years of age. The incidence of cancer, unlike those for heart disease and stroke, has risen over time, thus encouraging speculation that this disease may be a killer of last resort [24, p. 147]. There are environmental risks associated with cancer, particularly smoking and chemical exposure.

Osteoporosis weakens the bones by leaching them out, thereby causing them to be more porous. Among the elderly, particularly post-menopausal women, bone fracture associated with falls is a serious physical threat that often results in disability and death. The implication of hip fracture for long-term care demands is radical. The physiological processes associated with bone loss have to do with the presence of reproductive sex hormones. As estrogen falls off after menopause, the replacement of this hormone can slow bone loss for women. Consistent and moderate exercise and calcium supplementation can also retard bone loss. A bone scan at menopause, and occasional scans later with attention focused on bone loss, could go a long way toward reducing the incidence of hip fractures among older women [41].

As should be noted about this brief review of chronic diseases, standard medical remedies have limited impact. On the other hand, more holistic strategies seem to be effective in slowing the effects of aging. Specifically, persons can take an active, even proactive, role in fostering health. Lifestyle changes, for example, can go a long way toward enhancing the quality of a person's existence. But typically this *modus operandi* is kept ancillary to medical treatment, or is considered to be something idiosyncratic. Such behavior is not considered by most physicians to be indicative of a general medical regimen. As a result, this activity will not likely be viewed by traditionalists as the cornerstone of a public medical policy.

INTERVENTIONS AND OLD AGE

Each successive birth cohort of older persons is different from the previous ones. But what is happening to younger cohorts will probably be reflected in the future among the elderly. James Fries reports in a 1989 summary that since 1953, tobacco consumption has declined in the United States by 40 percent, as has the use of butter (by 1/3), whole milk and cream (by 1/4), and saturated animal fats for cooking (by 40%) [42].[10] He further reported that during the same period, vegetable and fish consumption increased. Population studies show that these behavioral changes have had strong statistical associations with lower morbidity, and, as a result, with the potential reduction in the use of health services and with producing longer life.

Furthermore, Manton and his colleagues demonstrate, for example, that chronic disability prevalence among community-dwelling and institutionalized persons over sixty-five years of age declined 4.7 percent

[10]Citing Fries and others, Fox also discusses the behavioral changes that could produce strong cohort health effects in the future.

between 1984 and 1989 for those over the age of sixty-five. The probability of avoiding disability over the 1984-1989 period increased with age, so that the declines in chronic disability prevalence were greatest among those over age eighty-five [43]. If there were to be a 5 percent decline in disability among the elderly for several additional five-year periods, this trend would substantially alter the long-term care needs in this population in the next century. But until this happens, no one should count on continued large declines. The point is that these declines may be the delayed benefits of lifestyle changes, such as those noted by Fries during the past thirty years. If so, these gains would signal another victory of environmental and holistic medicine. Manton and his collaborators speculate that these improvements may be due to higher levels of education and income in the later elderly cohorts, as compared with earlier ones. Higher educational attainment and income contribute to a greater understanding of the dietary and lifestyle factors that influence health and well-being. This line of reasoning is also supported by the work of Maddox and Clark, who found a strong negative association between both education and income and disability rates [44].

Higher educational and income levels of successive cohorts of elders, along with lifestyle changes and increases in preventive medicine, suggest that chronic disability rates will continue to decline. Although such improvements would be welcomed, modest declines in disability prevalence in the late 1980s will not be enough to offset the growth of the elderly population. The absolute numbers of the chronically disabled will certainly continue to expand, for only so much can be done to forestall the effects of population aging.

Nonetheless, what kinds of medical attention can be given to patients with chronic illness other than representative of biomedicine? 1) On the front end, more medical research should be aimed at issues related to prevention. 2) Behavior that brings down risk factors associated with chronic disease should be supported with medical dollars. 3) Information should be provided to help family caregivers to locate rehabilitation therapists, equipment, and services for the patient in their care. Additionally, more resources should be provided for the outright support of informal caregivers, for example, through respite and adult day care. Ideally, these services should be part of managed care systems. 4) Psychological counseling and support group referrals should be supported during the critical and transitional phases of chronic care. 5) Training should be emphasized in coping strategies that are important for adequately managing symptoms. And 6) home health nursing, home use equipment, and instrumental support should be given serious attention, so that patients can be maintained in their communities.

Each of those factors have proven to be helpful in the care of chronically ill persons [45]. Moreover, those kinds of interventions are cost-effective, and definitely less expensive than alternative biomedical interventions. But are these modes of treatment scientific, high-tech, or even capable of the formalization sought by most physicians? From the biomedical perspective, those modes of treatment may even be viewed as a return to a by-gone era. These relatively low-tech approaches seem more representative of the seventeenth than the twentieth century. Any why would physicians want to return to this dismal period of medicine?

CONCLUSION

Most of the diseases that will eventually afflict Americans cannot be cured, although the impact of these maladies can be postponed through preventive medicine and lessened through skillful management. Prevention, however, along with health promotion, is viewed in biomedicine as the province of public health, involves activities conducted primarily by nurses and social workers, and requires resources that lie outside of the bailiwick of the medical profession. Keeping the present course, however, will likely be disastrous financially and harmful to patients. Pre-clinical conditions will be ignored until they pass the clinical disease threshold, and diagnoses will be made that are appropriate for acute problems. How can this be viewed as good medical practice?

Unfortunately for the medical establishment, this strategy has become too expensive for the patient, employer, and government to afford to continue to support, and has cost medicine its special relationship with business. Biomedicine must adapt or die. The problem is that adaptation, at this time, requires that a broader perspective on health and healing be adopted. For this to happen, the biomedical model must be placed in a new context. Stated simply, the epistemology of medicine must be expanded, thereby fostering the development of a wider range of possible interventions. In this way, medicine can become more amenable to the complexity of chronic illness; medicine can meet the challenges of a new social environment.

Many physicians, however, are not ignorant about the problems that will be posed for medicine by the increase in chronic illness. In fact, chronicity is now a hot topic. Having to cope with chronic diseases has generated an uneasiness among physicians, because of the narrow approach that has been taken to complex medical problems. Many physicians feel trapped by their paradigm and are aware of the advantages that the broader models used by holistic, environmental, and behavioral medicine have over their own. Physicians are continuously reminded of the limitations of the biomedical model. Nonetheless, the conditions have not been established for a new paradigm to arise. The proper framework has not been developed that is required to foster the expansion of medicine.

In the rush to formulate a national health care plan, the context of practice should not be overlooked. For the most part, however, attention has been directed to the logistics of reform. Yet without rethinking the paradigm of medicine, old ideas are likely to be recycled. And because this new plan should reflect changes in the social environment, especially the aging of the population, such as rehash of issues is extremely disappointing. But scrutiny of the traditional medical paradigm is not usually a serious part of planning. This failing must be rectified if medicine is to be socially responsive!

In the next chapter, an attempt will be made to describe what such an alternative paradigm would look like. Such a paradigm would have to be appropriate to the treatment of chronic disease, not just in its acute later stages, but in its pre- and early clinical condition. In addition, the new paradigm would have to treat the patient as a person, who has both a mind and a body and exists in social and physical contexts. Furthermore, these nonphysiological factors would have to be viewed as linked inextricably to health and illness. This paradigm shift would thus be striking, and support a completely different kind of health care. This new system may appear strange at first to health professionals and physicians, but, nonetheless, will be properly attuned to the changing needs of the population. Perseverance may be needed to appreciate the wisdom of this shift, along with a willingness to abandon the presuppositions and limitations of a familiar philosophy.

REFERENCES

1. D. Fox, *Power and Illness: The Failure and Future of American Health Policy,* University of California Press, Berkeley, 1993.
2. S. J. Reiser, *Medicine and the Reign of Technology,* Cambridge University Press, Cambridge, pp. 174-195, 1978.

3. L. H. Garland, On the Scientific Evaluation of Diagnostic Procedures, *Radiology, 52,* 1949.
4. L. G. Davies, Observer Variation in Reports on Electrocardiograms, *British Heart Journal, 20,* pp. 153-161, 1958.
5. J. S. Butterworth and E. H. Reppert, Auscultatory Acumen in the General Medical Population, *Journal of the American Medical Association, 174,* pp. 32-34, 1960.
6. D. Follmann, M. Wu, and N. L. Geller, Testing Treatment Efficacy in Clinical Trials with Repeated Binary Measurements and Missing Observations, *Communications in Statistics: Theory and Methods, 23,* p. 557ff., 1994.
7. A. H. Wu, S. S. Wong, K. G. Johnson, J. Callies, D. X. Shu, W. E. Dunn, and S. H. Wong, Evaluation of the Triage System for Emergency Drugs-of-abuse Testing in Urine, *Journal of Analytic Toxicology, 17,* pp. 241-245, 1993.
8. H. P. Stapp, *Mind, Matter and Quantum Mechanics,* Springer-Verlag, New York, pp. 37-45, 1993.
9. L. Foss and K. Rothenberg, *The Second Medical Revolution: From Biomedicine to Infomedicine,* Shambhala, Boston, 1987.
10. W. C. Menninger, Psychiatric Experience in the War: 1941-1946, *American Journal of Psychiatry, 103,* p. 578, 1946.
11. J. Kiecolt-Glaser, R. Glaser, E. C. Strain, J. C. Stout, K. L. Tarr, J. E. Holliday, and C. E. Speicher, Modulation of Cellular Immunity in Medical Students, *Journal of Behavioral Medicine, 9,* pp. 5-21, 1986.
12. P. E. S. Freund and M. B. McGuire, *Health, Illness and the Social Body: A Critical Sociology,* Prentice Hall, Englewood Cliffs, New Jersey, 1991.
13. K. B. Alster, *The Holistic Health Movement,* The University of Alabama Press, Tuscaloosa, p. 104ff., 1989.
14. P. Mattson, *Holistic Health in Perspective,* Mayfield Publishing Co., Palo Alto, California, 1982.
15. J. B. McKinlay and S. M. McKinlay, The Questionable Contribution of Medical Measures to the Decline in Mortality in the United States in the Twentieth Century, *Milbank Memorial Fund Quarterly/Health and Society, 55,* pp. 405-428, 1977.
16. A. Anderson, How the Mind Heals, *Psychology Today,* 1982.
17. P. Starr, *The Social Transformation of American Medicine,* Basic Books, New York, 1982.
18. R. Zaner, *Ethics and the Clinical Encounter,* Prentice Hall, Englewood Cliffs, New Jersey, 1988.
19. D. Chopra, *Unconditional Life,* Bantam Books, New York, pp. 10-15, 1991.
20. F. M. Frohock, *Healing Powers,* The University of Chicago Press, Chicago, pp. 23ff., 1992.

21. J. M. Mitchell and E. Scott, New Evidence of the Prevalence and Scope of Physician Joint Ventures, *Journal of the American Medical Association, 268,* pp. 80-84, 1992.
22. D. J. Rothman, *Strangers at the Bedside: A History of How Law and Bioethics Transformed Medical Decision Making,* Basic Books, New York, 1991.
23. President's Commission, *Deciding to Forego Life-Sustaining Treatment,* Washington, D.C., 1983.
24. M. Mittelmark, The Epidemiology of Aging, in *Principles of Geriatric Medicine and Gerontology,* edited by W. Hazzard, E. Birman, J. Blass, W. Ettinger, and J. Halter (eds.), McGraw Hill, New York, pp. 135-151, 1993.
25. S. Katz, Assessing Self-maintenance: Activities of Daily Living, Mobility and Instrumental Activities of Daily Living, *Journal of the American Geriatrics Society, 31,* pp. 721-727, 1983.
26. M. Neal, C. Pratt, and E. Schafer, *Aging Oregonians: Trends and Projections, 1993,* Oregon Gerontological Association, Portland, Oregon, 1993.
27. J. A. Lueck-English, *Health in the New Age,* University of New Mexico Press, Albuquerque, 1990.
28. W. G. Weissert, Rationale for Public Health Insurance Coverage of Geriatric Day Care: Issues, Options, and Impacts, *Journal of Health Politics, Policy and Law, 3,* pp. 555-567, 1979.
29. B. D. Dunlop, Need for and Utilization of Long-term Care among Elderly Americans, *Journal of Chronic Disability, 29,* pp. 75-87, 1993.
30. W. J. McAuley and R. Blieszner, Selection of Long-term Care Arrangements by Older Community Residents, *The Gerontologist, 25,* pp. 188-193, 1985.
31. R. Avery, A. Speare, Jr., and L. Lawton, Social Support, Disability and Independent Living of Elderly Persons in the United States, *Journal of Aging Studies, 3,* pp. 279-293, 1989.
32. C. C. Saltz, E. B. Palmore, R. Valez, K. Magrudere-Habib, and R. Uhlig, Alternatives to Institutionalization: Estimates of Need and Feasibility, *Journal of Applied Gerontology, 32,* pp. 137-149, 1983.
33. D. L. Rabin and P. Stockton, *Long-term Care for the Elderly: A Factbook,* Oxford University Press, New York, 1987.
34. National Center for Health Statistics, Characteristics of Nursing Home Residents, Health Status, and Care Received: National Nursing Home Survey, U.S., 1977, *Vital and Health Statistics, No. 92,* Public Health Service, Hyattsville, Maryland, 1983.
35. B. J. Soldo, In-home Services for the Dependent Elderly, *Research on Aging, 7,* pp. 281-304, 1985.
36. C. S. Kart and R. E. Dunkle, Assessing Capacity for Self-care among the Aged, *Journal of Aging and Health, 1,* pp. 43-45, 1989.

37. U.S. Senate Special Committee on Aging, the American Association of Retired Persons, the Federal Council on the Aged and the U.S. Administration on Aging, *Aging America: Trends and Projections,* U.S. Government Printing Office, Washington, D.C., 1991.
38. C. F. Longino, Jr., B. J. Soldo, and K. G. Manton, The Demography of Aging, in *Gerontology: Perspectives and Issues,* K. F. Ferraro (ed.), Springer Publishing Co., New York, pp. 19-41, 1990.
39. P. M. Becker and H. J. Cohen, The Functional Approach to the Care of the Elderly: A Conceptual Framework, *Journal of Geriatrics and Gerontology, 32,* pp. 923-929, 1984.
40. K. G. Manton and B. J. Soldo, Health Status and Services Needs of the Oldest Old: Current Patterns and Future Trends, *Health and Society, 63,* pp. 286-319, 1985.
41. R. Lindsay and F. Cosman, Primary Osteoporosis, in *Disorders of Bone and Mineral Metabolism,* F. L. Coe and M. J. Favus (eds.), Raven Press, New York, pp. 831-886, 1992.
42. J. F. Fries, The Compression of Morbidity: Near or Far? *Milbank Memorial Fund Quarterly/Health and Society, 67,* pp. 208-231, 1989.
43. K. G. Manton, L. Corder, and E. Stallard, Changes in the Use of Personal Assistance and Special Equipment from 1982 to 1989: Results from the 1982 and 1989 NLTCS, *The Gerontologist, 33,* pp. 168-176, 1993.
44. G. L. Maddox and D. O. Clark, Trajectories of Functional Impairment of Later Life, *Journal of Health and Social Behavior, 33,* pp. 114-125, 1992.
45. G. H. De Friese and A. Womert, Informal and Formal Health Care Systems Serving Older Persons, in *Aging, Health, and Behavior,* G. Ory, R. P. Ables, and P. D. Lipman (eds.), Sage, Newbury Park, California, pp. 57-82, 1992.

CHAPTER
6

The Emerging Paradigm

As has been mentioned throughout this book, biomedicine is not flexible enough to handle many of the chronic problems that are part of becoming old. Or, perhaps more important, these issues are dealt with narrowly and thus improperly by the biomedical model. The chronicity associated with many of the ailments experienced by the aged defy the restrictive analysis offered by biomedicine. These problems are not "context-free," and therefore cannot be fit into the neat biochemical, mechanistic, cause-effect scheme most physicians prefer [1, p. 47].

In the case of the aged, the distinction made by Kleinman, Eisenberg, and Good between disease and illness is particularly relevant [2]. As persons grow old, chronic and degenerative problems become paramount. Nonetheless, these issues cannot be classified accurately as diseases [3]. They do not have a precise moment of onset, do not have a single and unambiguous cause, do not have an end that can be modified, and are related to a melange of factors that are tied indirectly to physiology. Certain key requisite conditions, in other words, are not met. These diseases "call for an understanding of the interaction between the multiple variables in both the causation and course" of a problem, which is a demand that challenges the standard approach to biomedicine [2, p. 252]. This conclusion is obviously at variance with the biomedical model.

Rather, most of the difficulties encountered by older persons should be viewed as illnesses. At this juncture, Szasz's definition of mental illness as a "problem in living" is instructive [4, p. 8]. That is, many of the complaints raised by the aged pertain to their inability to perform as they did when they were younger, thereby spawning personal and interpersonal conflicts. In this sense, the experience of discomfort, or

illness, becomes especially germane, as opposed to simply the physiological side of functioning. As Good writes, illness is a "syndrome of
experience" [5, p. 5]. Aches and pains, for example, are related to
difficulties in managing their environment, family problems, emotional
crises, and a general malaise about growing old. With regard to illness,
physiology is understood to be implicated in a matrix of social and
cultural considerations. Illness is a problem that is a thoroughly cultural, or interpretive, issue. Illness exists only with regard to persons
trying to forge an existence.

As should be noted, illness is a much broader category than disease.
But because of the basic tenets of biomedicine, illness is equated with
disease. This misunderstanding is unfortunate for any population, but
particularly the aged. For as persons become older, the majority of
their problems tend to almost always violate the assumptions of the
biomedical model. Their physiology, in short, cannot be directly linked
to their problems, as many physicians tend to believe. Medicine's
"crisis" can, in part, be traced to this breakdown in dualism, which is
compounded by a refusal to be "concerned with psychosocial issues
which lie outside medicine's responsibility and authority" [6, p. 129]. As
a consequence of focusing mostly on bio-chemistry, patients begin to
feel dissatisfied with their treatment. However, this is not merely a
matter of misperception. Many of the difficulties experienced by the
aged are, in fact, unrelated or tangentially related to physiology.

Consistent with the position advanced by Pierre Bourdieu, illness
constitutes an experiential field [7, p. 96]. "To think in terms of field,"
writes Bourdieu, "is to *think relationally.*" Accordingly, as opposed to
disease, illness encompasses a variety of spheres; illness is multivalent
with respect to origin, cause, and remedy. Illness is implicated in a
wide range of emotional, cultural, and social factors. Required for a
proper diagnosis of illness, therefore, is a model that is far more open
than the one indicative of biomedicine. Indeed, mistaking illness for
disease may culminate in masking a variety of problems.

A paradigm is emerging, however, that is compatible with this
need for openness and sensitivity. *A priori* distinctions between
fact and value, truth and opinion, and center and periphery, for
example, are not a part of this viewpoint. Without a doubt, making
assumptions such as these can unduly truncate an investigation.
For example, a particular course of study can easily be regarded as
worthless, without a proper hearing. The usual approach to conceptualizing a problem—"one germ, one disease, one therapy"—may be
appropriate for understanding a disease, but not an illness [8, p. 58].

An illness is only partially physiological, and thus cannot be this neatly circumscribed.

Illnesses are manifested bodily, but do not have necessarily a physiological cause. Therefore, giving priority to the body as a primary causal variable is not warranted. When assessing an illness, the body must be placed in a much larger framework. Perhaps doctors would be more successful, writes Zola, if they had "the knowledge and awareness of the patient's views of health, sickness, his expectations and his reasons for seeking help" [9, p. 119]. Therefore, rather than a concatenated series of events, a field or constellation is better imagery for visualizing an illness. For the physiological body resides in an existential field that is not exhausted by any particular variable; the domination of one variable over others is never automatically assured in an illness.

Within this burgeoning paradigm, *a prioris* are referred to a "metanarratives" [10, p. xxiv]. Metanarratives are sources of information that are assigned a seignorial status, but are never reflected on critically. In the biomedical model many of these grand narratives are present. For instance, associating facts with physiological markers is not questioned. Furthermore, laboratory tests are accepted to be unbiased and objective. As a result, medically derived knowledge is elevated above all others throughout the intervention process. In this way, a hierarchy of knowledge is established that is imagined to be indisputable. To a great degree, medical knowledge becomes the canon for undertaking treatment.

But this monolithic world is beginning to break apart. In the arts, literature, philosophy, and even physical science finding a universal foundation, or *archē*, for knowledge and order is thought to be dubious [11]. The reason for this difficulty is quite simple: the dualism necessary to sequester this base from contingencies is no longer available. Deprived of this safe haven, all knowledge lies on a similar plane. No knowledge, in other words, can be called absolute, while everything else is deemed relative. This distinction cannot be maintained in the absence of the special location necessary to preserve unadulterated facts. Newton's primordial vision is thus replaced by a multiplicity of views, which, in their own terms, have validity [1, p. 144].

Sometimes this predicament is recognized to signal the onset of the quantum world, while at others this rejection of dualism is characterized as the "postmodern condition" [1, pp. 137-155]. In each case, however, reality is portrayed in a similar way. Specifically, "there is no absolute deterministic level of description" [1, p. 151]. What this means is that there are no innocent descriptions, or statements devoid of presuppositions. As Rorty writes, "there is no way to stand outside of all human needs and observe that some of them . . . are gratified by detecting 'objective sameness and difference in nature'" [12, p. 8]. Accordingly, a pure picture of reality is never acquired. All that is ever seen is a particular rendition of reality, which is framed in one way or another by an interested observer. For this reason, Habermas asserts that interests cannot be stripped from knowledge [13]. Reality is not simply a matter of perception, but invention.

Knowledge is thus decentered. As Gebser declares, the "center is everywhere" nowadays [14, p. 544]. Because a primordial core of reality cannot be justified, at best existence can be divided into different and competing spheres. One set of assumptions yields a particular reality, while a different cognitive map produces another. The implication is that any claim to be absolute does not have a physical basis. In the face of this collage of realities, giving precedence to one segment is a matter of convention. Any one can be chosen for this honor, but none can demand this recognition. Epistemological pluralism is the standard, and thus there is no room for the dogmatism that pervades the biomedical model.

Due to this dispersal of knowledge, there is no justification for starting an investigation in any single place, following a preconceived course, or expecting to end in a special location. Such rigidity is neither required nor allowed in a decentered world. This attitude is certainly compatible with the view that existence is comprised of multiple realities. In a decentered world, *a prioris* are replaced by direct experience as the appropriate place to inaugurate a search for knowledge. If canons do emerge, writes Fish, they should be recognized as a "response to historical needs and contingencies," rather than absolutes [15, p. 261]. Decentering knowledge, in other words, does not mean that valid data cannot be procured, but only that throughout a search for information the bounded and limited nature of any starting point must be recognized.

THE HUMAN LINK TO KNOWLEDGE

Basically, advocates of biomedicine are foundationalists. Foundationalists believe that "claims can be justified on the basis of some objective method" . . . , as opposed to the "accidents of education and experience" [16]. Applied to medicine, this definition suggests that a certain *modus operandi* has a seignorial status, while all others are not well substantiated and should be treated as frivolous. Certain methods, theories, and practices are unquestioningly valid, for they are justified by principles that exist *sui generis*. Hence biomedicine is not completely purged of metaphysics, for the practice of traditional medicine is underpinned by specific dogmatic commitments. Remnants of old-fashioned fundamentalism can thus be found at the center of the biomedical model.

To appreciate why foundationalism is undermined by post-modernists, their view of language must be understood. Borrowing from the later work of Wittgenstein, Lyotard argues that all knowledge is mediated by "language games" [10, pp. 9-11]. This is quite a radical position to take! As opposed to traditional theories of symbolism, Lyotard is saying that language does far more than "point to," "stand for," or "indicate" an objective reality. Rather, and directly related to rendering foundationalism passé, speech is recognized to have a pragmatic thrust. Reality, in other words, cannot escape from the grip of language, and thus the meaning of norms, laws, and rules has a linguistic cast.

Derrida makes this point with his now infamous declaration, "Nothing exists outside of the text" [17, p. 158]. There is no other side of language; there is no outside of language. Contrary to these dualistic conceptions, everything is mediated by language. Speech acts seep into every facet of life. There is no chance of escaping from the influence of language, in order to capture a glimpse at a pristine reality. All that can ever be known is an interpretation of reality. A so-called literal reading of the world is thus impossible. With a break from language ruled out, Roland Barthes announces that even "objectivity is only one image-repertoire among others" [18, p. 52]. No foundation can be invoked, accordingly, that does not reflect a consensus achieved through language use.

The zero or null point essential to foundationalism cannot be sustained [19, p. 13]. Language, instead, prescribes what is possible. Biomedicine, along with positive science, constitutes a language game. "Society is not only continually creating new diseases," notes Zola, "but constantly altering the forms of old ones" [9, p. 23]. These changes occur because the domain of biomedicine is organized around various definitions, conceptual schemes, imagery, and philosophical propositions. And once someone is inside of this web of discourse, reality assumes a particular form. But outside of this framework, the biomedical model may have little relevance. As a result, elevating biomedicine to the center of treatment is certainly open for discussion.

But perhaps more significant is that dualism is subverted. Presupposed by dualism is the ability to escape from subjectivity and encounter evidence divorced from interpretation. In this way, no illusions can be perpetrated about truth, for a reality is available for inspection by anyone who has the necessary time and skill. But Lyotard contends that "knowledge is no longer the subject, but in the service of the subject" [10, p. 36]. There is no subjectless knowledge, regardless of the claims made about objectivity.

But what about medicine becoming a value-free science? Nothing, but especially illness, can be examined in the impersonal way demanded by this kind of science. Because medicine invades the human soul, intimacy is required between the patient and practitioner [20, pp. 283-292]. Medicine is thus basically a moral enterprise, as opposed to a technical one. Required by this conclusion, however, is that many fundamental themes of biomedicine must be rethought. Specifically, these ideas must be given a human cast. They must be tied to human *praxis,* or the unique ability of persons to make and remake themselves and their surroundings, a perspective generally denied in biomedicine. Medicine must be redeployed with the awareness that the experiential and molecular levels are not the same. More to the point, every molecule is pervaded by experience that provides a person's existence with order and meaning. Dossey describes this to be a condition where the "microscopic world of atoms and molecules [is linked] to the world of human behavior" [21, p. 97]. Wherever knowledge is sought, the human element is integral to this process. Even in the most remote recesses of life, existential questions are operative. Medicine is no exception.

KÖRPER OR LIVED-BODY

At the end of his book *The Order of Things,* Foucault writes that "man is an invention of recent date. And one perhaps nearing its end" [22, p. 387]. Later on in his discussion of the "author effect," he argues that texts do not have authors [23]. At first, various critics considered these statements to be absurd. For clearly "man" has not disappeared from the earth, while common sense suggests that a book is written by someone. Has Foucault gone mad? As opponents of postmodernism remark, has Foucault's distaste for reality finally led him into a world of total illusion?

What he is doing, instead, is mounting an attack against one of the last manifestations of traditional metaphysics. In other words, he is challenging the usual attempt to provide the self with an indubitable anchor. *Pneuma, psyche, cognition, id,* and, more recently, the "true" or "real self" have been the designations used to secure a person's identity. Behind all the social veneer and myriad of conventions, individuals can feel confident that their existence is grounded in nature. Simply stated, the self is not evanescent, but substantial. Every person has essential traits, often referred to as a "human nature," that are purported to be universal.

Foucault is introducing the postmodern self. Accompanying the demise of dualism, the usual justifications for "man" are outmoded. Likewise, Lacan argues that "woman" no longer has a *raison d'être* [24]. Their point is that language also extends to the core of a person's identity, and thus searching for inherent characteristics to legitimize the self is futile. As existentialists are fond of saying, there is no essence that precedes existence. There is nothing lurking within the interstices of *praxis* that guarantees the perpetuation of a self. Barthes summarizes the arrival of this diaphanous self when he states that the "I is nothing other than the instance of saying I" [25, p. 145]. Within the nuances of speech is where the self resides.

In the postmodern world the self is made, but not in a deterministic manner. Postmodernists "insist on the *indeterminacy of the body*" [26, p. 80]. While other persons and environmental factors are involved in the development of the self, interaction with them is not monological or one-directional. Although the self is not created in isolation, these outside considerations do not simply impinge on the individual like stimuli. Because interaction with a person, place, or event, for example, is mediated by interpretation, these elements are referred to by postmodernists as imaginary [27]. By this is meant that another person's actions are interpretive rather than real. And even when a correct understanding of the other's behavior or an event is acquired, this so-called common reality is simply a shared mode of interpretation.

But what about the impact of institutions on the formation of the self? Encounters with these entities are usually thought to be more formidable than with regular persons. Individual behavior may be interpretive and thus contingent, but institutions are typically believed to be impregnable. As a consequence of postmodernism, however, institutions are not divorced categorically from persons and the symbolism that pervades an individual's identity. In short, institutions are also mediated by language use. Therefore, to paraphrase Schutz, institutions represent an agreement not to question a particular set of behavioral expectations. He refers to this maneuver as the "epoché of the natural attitude" [28, p. 229]. In more postmodern parlance, institutions are linguistic habits, or interpretations that have gained longevity. Rather than a reality *sui generis,* institutions embody a collective fantasy.

The foundation of both the self and institutions consists of piling interpretations on top of one another, with no hope of reaching an uninterpreted *terminus.* And only through human intervention can this regression be brought to a halt. Persons are thus confronted by the *mise en âbime,* or abyss, postmodernists claim haunts the human condition. At this juncture one of Sartre's famous refrains comes to mind, which states that persons are condemned constantly to remake their destiny. Without the usual metaphysical props, there is no alternative.

But what does this talk about a postmodern self have to do with the body? Gabriel Marcel answers this question by noting that persons do not "have" bodies [29]. They do not possess their bodies like they do objects. A human body, he contends, is not an instrument that persons use. Rather than a possession, the body is an experiential field. Persons, in short, are incarnated as their bodies.

Marcel's point is that the body is not an autonomous thing. A possession is something that individuals covet, own, manipulate, and, possibly, dispose of when it breaks. Implied is a sense of distance between an owner and his or her possessions. But persons are not separated from their bodies; they do not hold their bodies at arms length, so to speak. Instead of disembodied, persons are revealed in the flesh. In fact, postmodernists believe that a person's identity is written through the body [30].

The body is neither a frame that constrains the spirit nor an object that responds to external prodding. Both versions are dualistic and sever the body from interpretation. The body, instead, is an "animate organism," which is enlivened by the same factors that give meaning to life [31, p. 49]. As mediated thoroughly by interpretation, the *soma* is a "lived body." The body is an existential construct. "The lived body," contends Leder, "is not just one thing *in* the world, but a way in which the world comes to be" [32, p. 25]. The lived body is the incarnation of a person's approach to life. Writers such as Ludwig Binswanger refer to the body as a mode of being-in-the world.

Beauty, pain, or imbalance, accordingly, is not simply a property of physiology. These traits may be tied to the physical body, but their meaning lies elsewhere. Their significance is derived from the social class, cultural, and gender issues, for example, that inundate the body. For as Merleau-Ponty describes, the body is a "chiasm"—"the field of the sensible world as interior-exterior"—that represents the embodiment of various modes of interpretation [33, p. 234]. The activity of the mind, as revealed in culture or gender, includes a bodily component. Hence mind-body dualism is generally defunct, and not simply in cases that physiologists cannot solve. The body is always "conscience-incarnee," or consciousness incarnate [31, p. 134]. The coordination of the body, therefore, transcends the realm of the physical.

The body is thus an expression; "the physiological [is] always intertwined with, and an expression of, the body's intentionality" [32, p. 28]. And if an intervention is going to be effective, this expressiveness must not be violated. The *meaning* of the body must be respected, or the personal or social significance of an illness will be missed. Accordingly, any so-called physical marker should be recognized as an intentional correlate of conscious activity. If this advice is heeded, medicine will have a socially responsible direction. The practice of medicine will take place within the region deployed as the body, instead of the abstraction known as physiology.

THE COPERNICAN REVOLUTION

Advocates of biomedicine want to return to a time prior to the work of Kant. Consistent with Hobbes, Locke, and Hume, and more recent empiricists who want to ignore Kant's revolution, the biomedical model has objectivity as its goal. Physicians are supposed to attend to facts and nothing more; empirical indicators and the laws of biochemistry are supposed to be the focus of attention. Proponents of this philosophy insist that, under the proper conditions, the mind will merely reflect reality. Unencumbered by subjectivity, a clear picture of empirical data can be obtained.

Despite this scenario, Kant claims that Hume awakened him from his dogmatic slumber. But what could Kant learn from Hume, for they hold diametrically opposing views on the philosophical spectrum? Actually, what Kant is saying is that Hume reinforced his position. Without the organizational activity of the mind, argues Kant, the world would be disjointed and chaotic. Described in terms of empirical indicators, reality would be atomistic and have no organization.

Kant's conclusion is quite straightforward. Empiricists believe that facts consist of discrete pieces of data, nowadays referred to as information "bits," that are imprinted on the mind. One piece follows another, with the mind marking their arrival. However, the mind is allegedly passive during this process, which, according to Kant, presents an insurmountable problem. Specifically, how can separate sense impressions be said to represent a series, montage, or any other pattern? Given only this sort of input, reality could not form a coherent whole. All that could be known are individual impressions, which would have a random distribution.

For this reason, Kant called for his now famous epistemological reversal. Because the world cannot be discovered among disparate sense data, reliable knowledge could not be forthcoming from strictly empirical indices. To have any understanding of the world, persons would have to be viewed as more than "somatic-sensory" beings [34, p. 100]. They would have to be able to regulate sense impressions, or the world would remain fragmented. As a result, Kant proclaimed that the mind must be actively involved in shaping reality, for existence does not consist of "the random dance of molecules" [35, p. 248]. The organizational capacity of the mind, stated simply, cannot be extricated from whatever is known.

Adhering to this anti-dualistic tradition, Husserl proclaimed that all knowledge is intentional. He defines intentionality as follows: "consciousness is always consciousness of something" [36, p. 13]. With this seemingly trite phrase, he undercut the Cartesian tradition. The mind is not an abstraction, as Kant could be interpreted as saying, which out of necessity has to intervene in the world. But instead, everything that is known is assumed to be tied inextricably to conscious activity. Consciousness and the world are never separate; the mediational effects of the mind can never be abridged. This awareness spawned by Husserl laid the groundwork for the acceptance of the Wittgensteinian thesis that has been refined by postmodernists. In the place of consciousness is language that extends indefinitely, thereby inundating empirical reality.

Due to the pervasiveness of interpretation, referring to the world as empirical is dubious. Consequently, phenomenologists coined new language to describe reality. The term they chose is the *Lebenswelt*, or "life-world." Husserl defines the life-world as a "meaning construct" that embodies a "universal, ultimately functioning subjectivity" [37, p. 112]. The idea is that the world is not a composite of moribund sense data, but instead is alive and reverberates with human significance. As a life-world, reality consists of meanings that are constituted through conscious intentionality. Reality is divided into various complementary regions, assert postmodernists, that are based on different assumptions about facts, norms, truth, and so forth. Each of these realms is engendered through a *"pétite narrative,"* or selective definitions, that does not necessarily have unlimited applicability [10, p. 60].

Reality does not exist, but instead multiple realities. Furthermore, writes Schutz, each one operates according to a unique "stock of knowledge" [28, pp. 38-40]. This information pool is comprised of the assumptions, recipes, and information a socially competent person is supposed to know. Within a particular region, in other words, a unique rendition of reality has been enacted that every occupant is expected to have mastered. This is the situation Lacan is describing when he states that truth has nothing to do with empirical reality [38, p. 306]. Truth, like facts, is housed within a specific life-word; truth and facts are thematic. Each region is a "little universe" [39, p. 183].

Being enamored of empirical indicators, accordingly, does not bode well for accurately evaluating a patient. Given the intransigence of interpretation, consulting his or her life-world may be much more effective. In this way, each datum can be placed within its proper context, and be viewed, as Husserl comments, as "subject-related" [37, p. 326]. Rather than trying to meet the information demands imposed by an inner circle of medical specialists, Zaner argues that a patient should be examined in terms of his or her "own specific biographical situation and its distinctive values, attitudes, history, linguistic usages, and habits" [20, p. 34]. Experience and data are thus united, so that the social, cultural, or personal meaning of a fact can be grasped. If the aim of a physician is to pay attention to reality, how can introducing a patient's life-world into a diagnosis be detrimental?

CAUSES AND PRAXIS

Proponents of the biomedical model adopt a very old version of causality, although their view of the relationship between cause and effect is outlined in terms of eighteenth-century physics. Causes, stated simply, are physical events that collide with others to bring about certain results. A type of mechanical chain reaction is thought to occur with one event following another in a logical sequence. Hence the designation A→B has become quite fashionable.

A cause precedes an effect. With regard to the onset of disease, a pathogenic agent invades an organism, thus disrupting the normal state of equilibrium. Furthermore, the association between A and B is not redundant, or instigated by another factor that is indirectly linked to A. The pathogen is the real cause, and not simply perceived to be related to a specific effect. Rather than a psychological phenomenon, this "generative theory of causation" reflects nature [40, pp. 62-65]. In other words, real events spawn equally substantial effects.

A cause supplies both the sufficient and necessary conditions to produce a specific outcome. This is where the theory of causality proposed by the early Greeks becomes relevant. These sages used the term *aition in a unique way,* when they discussed causality. For them, an effect owes its identity to a cause; the cause literally produces the effect. In more modern terminology, the cause serves as the necessary and sufficient precondition for a particular result. For all practical purposes, the cause is presumed to generate the result.

Most important for this discussion, the cause is autonomous. In a linear manner, a self-contained cause provides the impetus for an effect. Therefore, a cause is non-contingent, has inherent links to other events, and brings to fruition a predetermined end [1, p. 255]. Despite the desire to make modern physics scientific, the notion of causality sounds suspiciously religious. Nonetheless, a cause inaugurates and channels a series of events.

Placed in the medical context, a person's biological equilibrium is disrupted by a cause. In a purely physicalistic manner, the health of an organism is jeopardized. What is disconcerting about this scenario is that the individual is assumed to be passive. Presumed is the "intensity, frequency, direction, setting, validity, and evidence" about the cause [1, p. 254]. The person, accordingly, is locked within a framework—a matrix of forces—that cannot be influenced. In such a linear scheme, the effect does not act on a cause; a cause is not subject to manipulation. A cause is not involved in a dialogical, or two-way, relationship with an effect.

From a postmodern point of view, this portrayal of causality is too simplistic. First, a cause is not independent, but symbolic or linguistic. Prior to A leading to B, A must be interpreted. Subsequent to this act of interpretation, the potential of A can be assessed. Remember that nothing, even a cause, escapes untainted by language.

Second, variables are experientially, rather than simply statistically related. Consciously constituted assumptions, in other words, determine the probability of events, rather than abstract statistical curves. For example, within a particular language game the chances of an event occurring may be great, although statistically the likelihood of this effect arising may be very remote. A probability statement is a product of assumptions, but the issue remains which ones should be given credence? Postmodernists are clear about where their priorities lie—on the existential side. In other words, assumptions are not embedded in nature, but extend from certain choices that are made. Which assumptions are imagined to be true, accordingly, is a matter of preference. The presuppositions of the life-world subtend the abstractions of science. Therefore, the concepts used to organize daily life should not be overshadowed by the ideas adopted by scientists to explain events.

And third, a linear conception of the relationship between variables is inappropriate. But a circular model may also be insufficient. Because a person's life-world is not monolithic, more expansive imagery is required to capture the actual way in which variables are related. Most important is to recognize that variables form an expressive constellation, based on the themes that are operative in the life-world. While reflecting the work of Engel, Foss, and Rothenberg have used the neologism "biopsychocultural medicine" to describe this new model [1, p. 269]. Their point is that variables are not joined *a priori* in a mechanistic way. Themes change, priorities shift, and experiences occur that interject dynamism into conceptualizing causality.

Postmodernists, following the work of Weber, make a distinction between causal efficacy and cognitive significance. According to this differentiation, causal efficacy refers to the "norms of calculation or thinking, the correct solution to an arithmetic problem" [41, p. 230]. On the other hand, cognitive significance is the "subjective interpretation of a coherent course of conduct" [41, p. 230]. Clearly postmodernists favor the latter mode of analysis. The rationale for their choice is quite simple: people are not passive or trapped with an environment that dictates their behavior. Instead, through the exercise of language, a reality is socially constructed that serves to organize events.

A coherent course of conduct, therefore, is not a series of causes and effects that are linked in terms of mathematical probability. Rather, coherency is secured through the ability of persons to suture together experiences into a meaningful whole, which is described by some writers as a *Sinnzusammenhang* (a meaningful pattern). Within this montage, the old notion of cause is refurbished. Now a cause is understood to be deflected by *praxis* into a cultural milieu. A cause, stated differently, is something that gains attention because of its social significance and is viewed by persons as having relevance in a particular situation.

From a biocultural perspective, a "particular combination of biological, psychological, and cultural components, conditioned by certain environmental factors, forms the relevant unit of pathogenicity" [1, p. 279]. Without attempting to over sell the influence of the environment, the point is that pathogens exist within a social context. Rather than a simple relationship between cause and effect, factors such as diet, lifestyle, habit, and locale are vital in understanding pathology. In short, there are no simple proximate causes, at least from the perspective of postmodernism.

In the medical arena, this change means that persons do not simply wait to be attacked by an agent. They are busy making a life, which includes establishing the conditions necessary for a cause to have an effect. A host of factors, for example, may intervene and establish the conditions necessary for a disease to be viewed as a product of a cause. Therefore, a cause is simply a metaphor for a range of factors a person believes explains an event, or makes sense from a particular perspective. Due to this experiential foundation of causality, Perelman urges readers to differentiate rationality from reasonableness [42, pp. 117-123]. His argument is that a reasonable course of action reflects the interpretive mediation of cause and effect, while rationality does not. Rationality is thought to be universal and unencumbered by the life-world, because reason consists of the natural link between premises and conclusions [41, p. 230]. On the other hand, causality is reasonable, he claims, when the cause and effect make sense to those affected. In the end, uniformities are generated through the intervention of *praxis,* as opposed to abstract causes, a means that is not embroiled in nature. Ignoring this mediation will culminate in the isolation of causes that are personally and socially incomprehensible, although they may be statistically interesting. This seems to be the point Dubos is making with respect to comprehending the onset of sickness.

NORMS AND LOCAL DETERMINISM

What proponents of biomedicine have tried to accomplish is to dehistoricize norms. By appealing to a theory of equilibrium, contingency could be purged from norms. And with norms having a deep structure, to borrow from Chomsky, universal standards of medicine could be developed. Invariants could be proposed that transcend the limitations imposed by space and time.

Providing norms with this stability would certainly be beneficial for medicine. Discovering the one best way to treat a disease would be possible. Laws could be discovered that specify the most propitious approach to repelling a pathogen and rehabilitating a patient. Following these discoveries, medicine would have renewed validity and respectability. As Brown writes, "scientific medicine wrapped the modern doctor in an aura of therapeutic effectiveness" [43, p. 78]. The exalted status of medicine would thus be assured.

Sequestering norms from interpretation would preserve the ideology of medicine. Illness could be distinguished clearly from health; fact could be cleanly severed from illusion. As a result, a calibrated response can be made to a problem. Biomedicine could thus secure a monopoly over other remedies, for this approach is predicated on verifiable laws [43, p. 78].

Despite these claims, the laws of medicine cannot be removed from history. According to Gadamer, every attempt at understanding is subject to "effective history," "which determines in advance both what seems to us worth enquiring about and what will appear as an object of investigation" [44, pp. 267-268]. No viewpoint, stated differently, is final, complete, and representative of the end of history. All-encompassing knowledge cannot be procured, because every study is guided by certain prejudices, as he calls them, that form a horizon and dictate the type of questions asked and the answers considered to be relevant. Rather than ahistorical, norms always reside within a horizon of inquiry that is not permanent.

Postmodernists agree with this position. While borrowing from Thom, an original contributor to the popularity of catastrophe theory, Lyotard argues that norms are "locally determined" [10, p. 61]. Because of shifts in language use, reality is discontinuous. Different locations are constituted that may be only remotely related to others. Furthermore, crossing their boundaries may result in an encounter with a completely new reality. As opposed to smooth, reality is understood to be a jagged patchwork, a collage of competing views.

All norms are thus situated, or ensconced within particular patches. The norms that are the focus of biomedicine are no exception. These norms are not ultimately generalizable, simply because they are believed to be buried deep within the organism. This location is merely one among many where a norm can be lodged and not an Archimedean point. Normalcy, in this sense, cannot be separated from certain specifications. The question is no longer whether a state is normal, but rather which norm applies in a particular situation. Instead of homogenous, norms are heterogeneous. And any rendition of normalcy that becomes paramount, accordingly, is "agreed on . . . and subject to eventual cancellation" [10, p. 66].

The application of this idea to medicine is obvious. Normalcy cannot be appreciated when removed from personal expectations, cultural sanctions, and social goals. Rather than natural, all norms are political. Normalcy is political, writes Fish, because it "advance[s] or retard[s] someone's interests and declare[s] itself on issues in relation to which sides have already been chosen" [45, p. 251]. Through individual or collective cognitive acts, claims are advanced that elevate one viewpoint over another. The resulting arrangement is eventually adopted as normal. Acts of will are thus responsible for establishing the horizon of normalcy, as opposed to an abstract biophysical system.

Clearly in this debate over normalcy, physicians have taken charge. They have wrapped themselves in science and have claimed to have almost infallible insight into the human condition. Norms are thus defined by medicine. How persons feel, or should function, is defined by the medical establishment. Through public relations campaigns, and other means, the body has gradually come to be controlled by medicine. The body has thus become a political pawn. Through the use of various therapies and medicines, particularly drugs, true normalcy can be achieved. Most problematic, however, is that this medical viewpoint is presented to the public as reality, as opposed to an interpretation of normalcy. Due to their exaggerated claims, as remarked by Becker, physicians have become the moral entrepreneurs in modern society [46].

TECHNICAL EXPERTISE OR
COMMUNICATIVE COMPETENCE

Equating technical expertise with methodological rigor is supported by dualism. *Techne* is assumed to be autonomous and value-free, and thus able to put researchers into contact with an unadulterated reality. Presumed is that knowledge is objective and waiting to be discovered. Ensnaring data in an unbiased method, accordingly, is touted to be the best way to garner valid information.

Acquiring technical competence is thought to lead to truth. The mastery of technique is believed to produce the formalization and standardization necessary for this task. The subjectivity associated with the human element is thus controlled and unable to disrupt the knowledge acquisition process. In fact, the aim of this sort of science is to transform methodology into a mechanical affair. Step-wise instructions are adhered to that supposedly do not require interpretation. As a result, the image is created that a neutral conduit is available to channel data without any contamination.

The problem is that procedural refinement and improved technical sophistication do not necessarily result in increased accuracy. Under the guise of value neutrality, certain assumptions are often advanced that are incompatible with the region investigated. These are the tacitly held beliefs about objectivity, realism, linear causality, and so forth that sustain, for example, the culture of biomedicine. In the life-world where persons actually reside, however, these concepts may be irrelevant. But if knowledge is filtered through these ideas, a distorted picture of a particular social situation may be obtained. The public's views may be sacrificed, in order to become objective. Yet what passes for objectivity may be simply an irrelevant picture of reality, which is based on unverified values. Mills calls this version of science "abstracted empiricism" [47, pp. 50-75]. Because the focus on method obscures social life, his designation seems appropriate.

Due to the situated character of knowledge, becoming value-free can be counterproductive. What is to be gained by adopting a so-called universal perspective, when knowledge is local? In more medical terms, a standardized diagnostic scheme or well designed actuarial table may have scientific appeal, but they do not necessarily have widespread applicability. These and other formalized methods eventually run into problems that are spawned by the values operative in social life. A person's life-world does not disappear, simply because of a practitioner's desire to transcend values and become objective. Given the intransigence of the life-world, the methodology of a medical team should be value-relevant.

In Habermas' words, instead of technical expertise, the centerpiece of medical intervention should be "communicative competence." Rather than trying to achieve objectivity, understanding the "basic qualifications of speech and of symbolic interaction" should be a prime objective [48, p. 138]. What a medical practitioner should do, in other words, is to penetrate the pragmatic thrust of language. Gaining entreé to the language game that is operative in a person's life-world should be elevated in importance.

Each instrument that is used to gather information, therefore, should be approached as an invitation to dialogue. To reiterate, the purpose of methodology is not to eliminate values, but to encounter them in the right way, as Gadamer suggests. In this case, the right way consists of allowing definitions of risk, health and illness, and cure to be shaped by the life-world, as opposed to traditional medical protocol.

Knowing which assumptions apply and which do not has become a lost art. But by becoming conversant with these different presuppositions, and able to supply data with a proper context, communicative competence can be achieved. When this stage is reached, stories rather than data are recounted.

Neither the body, social indicators, nor environmental factors are divorced from the life-story of patients. The composite of these tales, moreover, constitute the life-world. Vital to comprehending these stories correctly, contends Barthes, is reading them in the way in which they were written originally by their authors [18, p. 189]. In medical practice, the author is the patient. As Cassell illustrates, however, learning how to read a patient's stories is not currently a key element of traditional medical education [49]. Physicians seem to be more interested in diagnosis and cure. But by focusing mostly on the disease state, a patient's story is unduly truncated; by not going beyond the parameters of the physical body, a patient's life is fragmented.

Reading a story correctly requires an open mind on the part of the physician. A plot must be followed, regardless of where it leads. Furthermore, transgressing the usual boundaries of medicine may be necessary, if a story is to make sense. Intelligibility, in this sense, has nothing to do with objectivity. Instead, making sense of a story has more to do with entering the world an author creates in a text. Again, as noted by Barthes, the story is a world, and not a fantasy that obscures reality [50, p. 84].

Sensitive reading, simply put, requires that the physician not be blinded by ideology. The promise of objectivity should not direct attention away from a patient's life-world. The denouement of a patient's story should not be distorted by preconceptions about scientific reasoning, or any other traditional beliefs about medical practice. Attaining communicative competence involves placing aside irrelevant values or prejudices, in order to grasp the personal and social identity persons are writing for themselves.

AVOIDING SYMBOLIC VIOLENCE

Avoiding symbolic violence is important to those who support this new paradigm. This particular sort of violence occurs when a person's experiences are undermined by a sign system. But repression that is carried out through signifiers is not often treated as violent. In fact, persons will regularly volunteer for the correctives that are suggested by medical authorities. They will do practically anything to acquire the physical features, emotional state, or social stature that is explained to be normal. What they do in the end is to replace their own experiences with expectations that are advertised as superior.

This repression is not recognized as violent because physical coercion is not involved. What happens is that persons become enamored of symbols—in the form of norms, role models, and personal or social traits—that are touted to epitomize normalcy, rationality, beauty, intelligence, and so forth [7, p. 168]. The reason why these characteristics are so attractive is that they are thought to reflect human ideals or universal standards. Because these traits have this exalted status, they are deemed worthy of veneration. The result of this idolatry, however, is that personal values are dismissed gradually as impediments to improvement.

Repression such as this can easily result from the uncritical use of the medical model. Associated with biomedicine is imagery pertaining to the body, development, health, and rehabilitation that can easily become hegemonic. Older persons, for example, can begin to engage in self-denial, in order to be considered normal according to these medical standards. With care directed to an idealized type, the actual person can be obscured. Instead of dealing with health, discussions mostly revolve around the question of adaptation and achieving a normal state [51]. As a result, the concrete individual becomes ancillary to fulfilling the mandates of a diagnostic scheme or therapeutic regimen. Returning the person to normal becomes more important than designing a socially sensitive and situationally appropriate intervention.

Such violence is averted by this new paradigm because medical ideals do not have a seignorial status. They are simply one way of constructing a patient's reality. The aim of this new strategy is to bypass these ideals and gain access to his or her experiences, to build a diagnosis from the ground up, so to speak. Accordingly, no one is cajoled into adjusting to norms that are at best irrelevant and at worst harmful. A patient is dealt with as a whole person, in a manner that recognizes his or her uniqueness. Instead of blinded by science and value-freedom, physicians become cooperatively involved with their patients in resolving a problem.

CONCLUSION

What this new thinking does is to undermine the unique status that is accorded biomedicine. Traditional medicine is placed in a new context, and illustrated to be a particular mode of framing medical problems. Furthermore, this strategy is not objective, but may actually subvert dealing with a patient in the most propitious way. Adhering to the preconditions prescribed by biomedicine may obscure a patient's real problems and restrict the search for remedies.

Subsequent to the anti-dualism announced by postmodernists, medicine is liberated from its former core. Medicine, in short, is placed in the midst of experience, and is revealed to be an experiential mode. As might be suspected, this change is quite dramatic; medicine is placed on entirely new footing. This is a framework that is new to both physicians and patients. Establishing experience as the center of medicine means that issues related to human existence guide care, rather than biomedical prerequisites.

In general, there is no longer any justification for the stranglehold biomedicine had on medical knowledge. As a result, medical inquiries can expand into areas that were formerly off limits. In this sense, holism may be pursued without fear of embarrassment on the part of either the patient or physician. Preferences of patients that were eschewed before can become an integral part of a treatment plan.

What patients have to say about their problem or themselves does not have to be accepted as ancillary to medical protocol. Communication, in short, does not have to be simply tolerated as a means to acquire objective data. Dialogue, instead, is an acceptable way, actually the only means, to discover the parameters of a patient's problems. And as part of this process, the goals, values, and overall orientation to life of a patient can be placed at the center of the medical record.

Patients no longer have to be severed from their bodies, divorced from their disease, and moved to the periphery of the treatment process, in order for an intervention to have the appearance of science. New levels of inclusion can thus be tried that were anathema to biomedicine. Theories of causality can be expanded to incorporate new and, possibly, strange variables, while serious attention can be given to treatments that were earlier pooh-poohed. Science can exist alongside alternative strategies, without fear of contaminating an intervention.

Given the nature of chronic disease, old persons will likely benefit from this expansion. But medicine in general will benefit from this move. As is discussed in the next chapter, medicine can be democratized. That is, every aspect of medical practice, even those most cherished, will be open for examination. As a result, medicine will become more socially responsive. And making medical practice more culturally relevant can only improve the currently strained relations between the public and practitioners. For every disease, not just chronic illness, can be dealt with better through increased sensitivity.

But as will be seen shortly, democratization can appear, at first, to be very radical. Moving the practice of medicine away from biomedicine has far-reaching consequences. Expanded inclusion means that ordinary persons are able to go where they were formerly not able to tread. The public is placed in a position to define illness, allocate resources, prescribe treatments, and outline the objectives of medicine. Clearly a new and likely frightening dawn is emerging for the medical establishment. Placing the citizenry at the core of medicine may be very threatening to those who want to keep medicine a closed society. But given the present state of medicine, this type of shake-up may be exactly what is needed.

As long as the traditional core of medicine is retained, nothing will change. The same old vested interests will be trying to promote their aims while the public suffers. The same experts, knowledge bases, and economic proposals will guide the application of medicine. In the end, care will be taken out of the hands of citizens, thereby making treatment less accessible and more likely to be irrelevant. And clearly, such a combination can hardly be expected to reduce the cost of care.

REFERENCES

1. L. Foss and K. Rothenberg, *The Second Medical Revolution: From Biomedicine to Infomedicine,* Shambhala, Boston, 1987.
2. A. Kleinman, L. Eisenberg, and B. Good, Culture, Illness, and Care, *Annals of Internal Medicine, 88,* pp. 251-258, February 1978.
3. J. H. Knowles, Introduction to 'Doing Better and Feeling Worse': Health in the United States, *Daedalus, 106*:1, pp. 1-7, 1977.
4. T. Szasz, The Myth of Mental Illness, in *Radical Psychology,* P. Brown (ed.), Harper & Row, New York, 1973.
5. B. J. Good, *Medicine, Rationality, and Experience,* Cambridge University Press, Cambridge, 1994.
6. G. L. Engel, The Need for a New Medical Model: A Challenge for Biomedicine, *Science, 196,* 1977.
7. P. Bourdieu and L. J. D. Wacquant, *An Invitation to Reflexive Sociology,* University of Chicago Press, Chicago, 1992.
8. J. H. Knowles, The Responsibility of the Individual, *Daedalus, 106*:1, 1977.
9. I. K. Zola, *Socio-Medical Inquiries,* Temple University Press, Philadelphia, 1983.
10. J.-F. Lyotard, *The Postmodern Condition: A Report on Knowledge,* University of Minnesota Press, Minneapolis, 1984.

11. J. W. Murphy, *Postmodern Social Analysis and Criticism,* Greenwood Press, Westport, 1989.
12. R. Rorty, *Objectivity, Relativism, and Truth,* Cambridge University Press, Cambridge, 1991.
13. J. Habermas, *Knowledge and Human Interests,* Beacon Press, Boston, 1971.
14. J. Gebser, *The Ever-present Origin,* Ohio University Press, Athens, 1985.
15. S. Fish, The Common Touch, or, One Size Fits All, in *The Politics of Liberal Education,* D. J. Gless and B. H. Smith (eds.), Duke University Press, Durham, 1992.
16. S. Fish, Pragmatism and Literary Theory, *Critical Inquiry, 11*:3, pp. 433-458, 1985.
17. J. Derrida, *Of Grammatology,* Johns Hopkins University Press, Baltimore, 1976.
18. R. Barthes, *The Grain of the Voice,* Hill and Wang, New York, 1985.
19. R. Barthes, *Writing Degree Zero,* Hill and Wang, New York, 1968.
20. R. M. Zaner, *Ethics and the Clinical Encounter,* Prentice Hall, Englewood Cliffs, New Jersey, 1988.
21. L. Dossey, *Space, Time, and Medicine,* Shambhala, Boston, 1982.
22. M. Foucault, *The Order of Things,* Tavistock Publications, London, 1970.
23. M. Foucault, What is an Author?, in *Textual Strategies,* J. V. Harari (ed.), Cornell University Press, New York, pp. 141-160, 1979.
24. J. Lacan, *Feminine Sexuality,* Norton, New York, pp. 137-148, 1982.
25. R. Barthes, *Image, Music, Text,* Hill and Wang, New York, 1977.
26. A. Weston, On the Body in Medical Self-Care and Holistic Medicine, in *The Body in Medical Thought and Practice,* D. Leder (ed.), Kluwer, Dordrecht, 1992.
27. M. Sprinker, *Imaginary Relations,* Verso, London, 1987.
28. A. Schutz, *Collected Papers, Vol. I,* Nijhoff, The Hague, 1962.
29. G. Marcel, *Being and Having,* Harper and Row, New York, 1965.
30. R. Jones, Writing the Body: Toward an Understanding of l'Ecriture Feminine, in *The New Feminist Criticism,* E. Showalter (ed.), Pantheon, New York, pp. 137-148, 1985.
31. R. M. Zaner, *The Problem of Embodiment,* Nijhoff, The Hague, 1964.
32. D. Leder, A Tale of Two Bodies, The Cartesan Corpse and the Lived Body, in *The Body of Medical Thought and Practice,* D. Leder (ed.), Kluwer, Dordrecht, 1992.
33. M. Merleau-Ponty, *The Visible and the Invisible,* Northwestern University Press, Evanston, 1968.
34. L. Landgrebe, *Major Problems in Contemporary European Philosophy,* Frederick Ungar, New York, 1966.
35. E. J. Cassell, The Body of the Future, in *The Body in Medical Thought and Practice,* D. Leder (ed.), Kluwer, Dordrecht, 1992.
36. E. Husserl, *The Paris Lectures,* Nijhoff, The Hague, 1975.

37. E. Husserl, *The Crisis of European Sciences and Transcendental Phenomenology*, Northwestern University Press, Evanston, 1970.
38. J. Lacan, *Ecrits*, W. W. Norton, New York, 1977.
39. W. Benjamin, *Reflections*, Harcourt Brace Jovanovich, New York, 1978.
40. H. Wulff, S. A. Pedersen, and R. Rosenberg, *Philosophy of Medicine*, Blackwell Scientific Publications, Oxford, 1990.
41. A. Schutz, *The Phenomenology of the Social World*, Northwestern University Press, Evanston, 1967.
42. C. Perelman, *The New Rhetoric and the Humanities*, D. Reidel, Dordrecht, 1979.
43. E. R. Brown, *Rockefeller Medicine Men*, University of California Press, Berkeley, 1979.
44. H.-G. Gadamer, *Truth and Method*, Crossroad, New York, 1982.
45. S. Fish, *Doing What Comes Naturally*, Duke University Press, Durham, 1989.
46. H. Becker, *The Outsiders*, The Free Press, Glencoe, Illinois, 1963.
47. C. W. Mills, *The Sociological Imagination*, Oxford University Press, London, 1967.
48. J. Habermas, Toward a Theory of Communicative Competence, in *Recent Sociology*, No. 2, H. P. Dreitzel (ed.), Macmillan, New York, 1970.
49. E. J. Cassell, *The Nature of Suffering and the Goals of Medicine*, Oxford University Press, New York, 1991.
50. R. Barthes, *Criticism and Truth*, University of Minnesota Press, Minneapolis, 1987.
51. M. Foucault, *The Birth of the Clinic*, Pantheon, New York, 1973.

CHAPTER
7

The New Paradigm and Public Policy

Many of the problems that are currently facing medicine result from dualism. The focus on technology, overuse of medication, clinical insensitivity, and waste can be linked to this philosophy. In order to be considered objective and scientific, physicians are removed farther and farther from their patients. After all, becoming objective requires that increased attention be paid to technical instruments, diagnostic schemes, recommended treatments, and actuarial tables, rather than to the desires and opinions of patients. With regard to the biomedical model, in short, integrating patient input into the intervention process receives low priority.

In this sense, dualism sets the stage for the alienation of patients. But some practical considerations are also involved in the current fusillade against medicine. The magic bullets to cure many diseases have not arrived. And given the chronic nature of the problems experienced by older persons, less emphasis will be placed on cure in the future [1, p. 82]. The etiological agent of these diseases cannot be assaulted in a direct manner, thereby insuring the rapid discovery of a cure. As a result, the mystique that has surrounded medicine will become increasingly difficult to maintain [2, p. 81].

The coming of age of baby boomers also poses problems for the medical establishment. This group has had a tendency to distrust authority, especially that which is unresponsive to persons. Furthermore, the interest in environmentalism expressed by this age cohort comes into conflict with the faith placed in chemicals by most physicians. And not to be overlooked is the health consciousness—vegetarianism, meditation, and exercise, for example—exhibited by many boomers. They tend to believe that persons should have control over their bodies, whether male or female [3, pp. 76, 121].

Furthermore, in the past few years, practically everyone has begun to question the economic side of the health care system. Care is gobbling up a greater slice of the gross national product every year. Indeed, those high in the medical hierarchy seem to be making more and more money, while everyone else worries about their jobs. Medical care has become a commodity that is sold to those who can pay the market price. Those who do not have medical insurance, accordingly, must avoid visiting a physician until the last minute. And when care must finally be sought, these unfortunate persons often find themselves in the second-tier of the health care system [4, pp. 17-21]. "A walk around our cities" claims Zola, "will often reveal how marginal are the facilities of municipal hospitals compared to the superior facilities of private voluntary ones" [5, p. 71].

Many of these complaints are not new. During the last half century, medicine has become especially elitist. But M.D.'s have never been trusted by everyone. Charges of exploitation have been leveled regularly against this profession. Their monopolization of health care, in short, has angered much of the population at one time or another [6, pp. 69-70].

What is new, however, is the schism that exists between many physicians and their patients. The so-called "bedside manner" of doctors, on the whole, has deteriorated over the years. At one time patients were treated more often as persons. But nowadays patients are clearly approached as objects and commodities. Due to the ubiquity of dualism, persons have become ancillary to their bodies. Practically every facet of their existence has been materialized and transformed into an object [1, p. 211].

With this deanimation of the clinical setting, criticism of biomedicine is very damaging. Formerly, these allegations could be tempered by the interpersonal contact between physician and patient. A human bond was present, in other words, that could allay the fears and suspicions of patients. But now this closeness has all but evaporated. Even when persons visit their family practitioner, their relationship is mediated by technical, bureaucratic, and professional considerations that increase patient dissatisfaction [7, pp. 189-207]. To be sure, distrust and animosity can easily fester and expand when interpersonal distance is encouraged and maintained.

The resulting alienation occurs at several levels. First, the knowledge base that guides intervention is abstract. Because primary consideration is given to scientific indices, the patient is systematically objectified. In fact, the entire medical enterprise is centered around special knowledge, which is presumed to be much more reliable than the opinions expressed by patients and ordinary people. The input that patients have into medical practice, therefore, is peripheral to the overall process of intervention [8, p. 89]. Alternatives to biomedicine may be available, but they are treated as unscientific and inferiorized.

Second, patients are not really partners with physicians in searching for a cure. Despite the public relations campaigns of the recent years—which tend to stress the need to communicate—reciprocity is not present [9, pp. 134-135]. The reason for this absence of dialogue is quite simple: patients do not have the information at their disposal required for the formation of a real partnership. Crucial knowledge is monopolized by the medical profession, and thus patients have little to contribute to their treatment. But before symmetry is possible between persons, the basis for equality must be established. In this case, medical knowledge must be disseminated throughout society. Once this occurs, the likelihood may be improved that widespread participation in the medical system will be a reality.

Third, accessibility to the centers of decision-making must be guaranteed to patients. For the most part, patients and most citizens are barred from the locations where most crucial decisions are made about health care. Corporate and hospital boardrooms, medical schools, and government offices, for example, are sanctuaries most persons never enter. But in these places deals are made that affect the health of the nation. Traditional seats of power, therefore, may have to be challenged before socially responsive medicine is possible.

Fourth, a wide range of principles should guide the practice of medicine, particularly in a diverse society such as the United States. Nonetheless, at this juncture, the so-called economic "bottom line" delimits most discussions about the delivery of health care. Economic incentives, for example, are considered to be the most important factors when considering change. As a result of this restriction, key elements of the present system must be preserved. Serious proposals about health care reform are thus prematurely truncated, because of the need to protect certain entrenched economic interests.

And fifth, certain assumptions have gone unchallenged pertaining to where valuable ideas originate. In this regard, the medical system has been turned over to a cabal of experts. These individuals have degrees, licenses, certificates, and training that gives them special privileges. Accompanying the acquisition of these accoutrements is the widespread belief that these persons are inherently smarter and more insightful than everyone else. Furthermore, with respect to questions of medicine, these experts are expected to dominate all discussions, without any criticism from patients. In fact, Berliner writes that "Their moral authority," in fact, "[has] reached well beyond the strict confines of medical practice" [10, p. 2]. Their influence has been extended far beyond their limited range of medical competence [11]. A sort of halo effect allows biomedical practitioners to dominate discussions and dismiss popular responses to medical issues as opinion.

In the end, a hierarchy is established, with patients and the general citizenry at the bottom. Hence the special status coveted by the medical establishment is defended. At this time, however, the power of conspiracy is diffused. Physicians have not had to threaten the public by withholding a vital service, for example, to get their way. Through a symbolic means, instead, most persons have been convinced that medical experts and other facets of the health care industry deserve their seignorial position. After all, physicians possess the knowledge and skills that are believed to be vital to the survival of persons. But when citizens have minimal control over their health, they are truly victims of the health care system; they are naive and ripe for exploitation.

Most persons dread becoming ill, have a meager understanding of the health care system, and panic when the bills begin to arrive. Clearly this is the way in which victims act. Their loss of control does not allow them to respond in a reasonable manner to illness. To transform the status of both patients and citizens, however, they must become fully informed about the intricacies of health care. In a word, the delivery of medical services must become democratized.

As should be noted, democracy is not necessarily viewed by traditionalists as a part of providing medical services. Therefore, the American populace will have to engage in some radical thinking about medicine, if a democratic medical institution is to be deemed desirable. Democratization cannot be said to exist, for example, simply because the shortcomings of physicians are sometimes reported in the press, the limitations of the biomedical model are acknowledged in some cases, and the public is encouraged to adopt healthy lifestyles. Even the ridicule that is heaped on American society for having so many uninsured citizens is not a sign democracy has arrived. These and other forms of criticism are often found in democratic polities, but in themselves do not constitute democracy.

As pointed out early on by Mannheim, democracy is sustained by a particular "spirit" or worldview [12]. This general outlook invites criticism, supports diversity, rewards creativity, and tolerates a multitude of goals. Democracy, in other words, does not constitute an ideology. Human action, or *praxis,* extends to the core of this system and gives it direction. Every position is tied to an interpretive framework that must compete for recognition. Consequently, there are no privileged viewpoints that must be protected, or the survival of the system will be threatened. In the place of metanarratives is radical pluralism; persons are not held hostage by absolutes and intimidated by other idols.

Anti-dualism is compatible with the need to democratize the culture of medicine. Following the rejection of dualism, human action pervades medical practice. Therefore, the exalted principles of biomedicine that reinforce hierarchy are defiled. Biomedicine, as discussed in the beginning of Chapter 3, becomes a symbolic system that must have personal or social confirmation for it to survive. Alienation is thus reduced, because the health care system is opened. Persons no longer have to be subordinated to images that undermine self-direction, individual insight, and their ability to make knowledgeable decisions about seeking treatment. But perhaps most important is that the so-called realities, economic or otherwise, that currently stifle change lose their appeal. There is nothing to prevent this society from charting a new direction, other than outmoded symbolism. As a sign system, the logic of medicine is open-ended. And in the absence of dualism, the symbolic impediments imposed by biomedicine can be easily overcome.

THE PROLIFERATION OF VIEWPOINTS

For most doctors, medicine and science are one in the same. The result is that the assumptions that sustain science channel the search for facts in medical practice. Data must have a particular appearance, adhere to well recognized patterns, and fit into prevailing theories before they are given any credence. Certain knowledge is thus regularly included in interventions, while other forms are systematically excluded. Without any investigation, select information is often presumed to be invalid because it does not conform to traditional mandates.

Most troublesome is that this esteemed stock of knowledge is considered to be objective. The data that fit into the strictures imposed by science are considered to be factual, due to their empirical nature. These pieces of information are procured in such a way that their validity is unquestioned. Because of the value-neutral posture of science, these data are unbiased and represent truth. Other knowledge, accordingly, is considered to be inexact.

Dualism allows an unfair comparison to be made between knowledge bases. Those that are associated with science are portrayed favorably, while all others are considered automatically to have serious flaws. Knowledge that is acquired through laboratory tests, experimentation, and clinical instruments is given primacy over soft data. Given this penchant for scientific rigor, information that is contaminated by the human element is usually dismissed as imprecise and unreliable.

Due to the widespread acceptance of dualism, the public is easily lulled into embracing this asymmetry between knowledge bases. For example, writes Carlson, "modern medicine has successfully isolated and denigrated nonallopathic practitioners and practice" [1, p. 72]. This task was relatively easy. After all, why would anyone seek out opinion and speculation, when sound scientific facts are available? Afraid of appearing to be irrational, the judgments of physicians are seldom jettisoned by the public, or challenged seriously by non-traditional practitioners. Questions may be raised, but real confrontations are rare. Citizens may be momentarily upset with the medical establishment, yet business as usual is not threatened. What other outcome should be expected, when objectivity is juxtaposed to subjectivity in this way?

Nonetheless, democratization must extend to knowledge bases, if medicine is ever to become socially attuned. All forms of information, at least initially, must be viewed as equal. For *a priori* distinctions about reason and objectivity only restrict unfairly input into medical decision-making. As might be suspected, so-called subjectivity is inferiorized and designated as speculative. With respect to patients, this approach to knowledge is disastrous. Simply put, because most patients are not scientific, their insights are disregarded. Likewise, the status of alternative remedies is questionable, because of their lack of a scientific grounding. But in the absence of a thorough discussion, why should certain views be treated as innately inferior to others? With science identified as uniquely objective, however, the manipulation of patients by physicians should be expected.

Yet once dualism is abandoned, nothing is objective. The source of true knowledge is not autonomous and unaffected by the human mind. In the absence of dualism, all information is interpretive and placed on an identical plane. A symmetrical relationship, accordingly, is present between knowledge bases. With regard to this condition, "multiple realities" can be said to exist [13, pp. 229-234].

This leveling of information is consonant with the democratization of knowledge. Only through discussion can one knowledge base become dominant, for there is nothing inherent to particular data that make them attractive. No mode of interpretation can demand such respect. If certain assumptions about health and illness had not been adopted, the biomedical model would not make much sense. What has occurred, writes Schutz, is that priority has been given to a particular collection of ideas, thereby enabling them to become a paramount reality. "Many sub-universes of reality of *finite provinces of meaning*" can be identified, claims Schutz, "upon which we may bestow the accent of reality" [13, p. 230].

One knowledge base is elevated over another through *praxis*, as opposed to the intercession of a divine or natural force. The current dominance of biomedical knowledge, in other words, is the product of specific social agreements. Allopathic medicine was funded, for example, rather than homeopathic [10, pp. 76-91]. Germ theory was supported, instead of social medicine. Key decisions have been made, which reflect political influence more than hard evidence, that resulted in biomedicine coming to dominate medical schools, hospitals, and clinics. In many instances, the idiosyncrasies of rich and powerful benefactors dictated the course of medical practice. These events were instrumental in the social constitution of the knowledge base that thrust biomedicine into the limelight. Accordingly, these political maneuvers sustained science and its claims about rationality and objectivity.

Subsequent to the demise of dualism, however, all knowledge bases are able to flourish. What were formerly thought to be inherent limitations to some plans are revealed to be interpretive and arbitrary. Hence there is no ultimate reality, which has the latitude to condemn other viewpoints to the status of opinion, idealistic rhetoric, or error. Labels such as these have relevance only after a position has been assessed in terms of particular goals, resources, contexts, and so forth. These contingencies, furthermore, are also determined through debate. Priorities can be renamed, due to the elimination of external constraints. For in a postmodern world reality is indeterminate, for "it is creative and original—organization is always unforeseeable" [14, p. 18]. In other words, what becomes normative is a result of choice, intimidation, or some compromise.

The insight offered by patients is thus able to compete with medical opinion for recognition. In this regard, Zola writes that "the increasing use of illness as a lever in the understanding of social problems represents no dramatic shift from a moral to an objectivity neutral view, but merely to an alternative strategy" [5, p. 282]. Accordingly, new options can be tried, without the stigma applied by advocates of biomedicine. New visions can be examined in their own terms, minus the bias conveyed by the biomedical model. Finally, ideas outside of biomedicine can receive a fair reading, and the public can ascertain their relevance.

DIALOGIC INTERVENTION

Currently, health care is predominately "physician-centered" [6, p. 5]. Decisions related to diagnosis and treatment are mostly within the purview of the medical team. Here, again, asymmetry exists between the physician and patient. Not only do doctors have a research base that is largely unquestioned, but they operate with almost complete immunity as experts. As a result, patients are rendered passive throughout the treatment process.

Evidence gathered during the past few years has shown that intervention is more successful when rapport is developed between a patient and physician [15, pp. 131-150]. Nonetheless, the presence of true dialogue between these parties is rare. Physicians have accumulated a body of knowledge that they share only reluctantly with the general public. More to the point, they have tried to restrict access to this information [16, p. 87]. Furthermore, as specialists, their skills are understood to have become refined over the years. And once someone has gained the title "expert," his or her judgments are accepted almost as a matter of faith. Supported by modern technology and other improved paraphernalia, the opinion of physicians is given a new aura of respectability.

Under this condition, how are patients and physicians supposed to be partners in seeking a cure to a problem? By the time a physician is contacted, patients are usually frightened. This combined with a lack of knowledge and the prestige of the physician, places a patient in a very vulnerable position. Yet becoming a full partner or ally in treatment requires more equality among the relevant parties than is currently the case. Partnership, according to Habermas, requires "the *public* practice of a shared, reciprocal taking over of perspectives" [17, p. 251]. Clearly, the relationship between the physician and patient can reach this plateau only be changing dramatically and becoming dialogical.

Individualism and autonomy are essential to forming a *bona fide* partnership [18, pp. 22-24]. Persons, in short, must be free to enter into this type of relationship. But this stipulation can be met only by eliminating the conditions that promote coercion and manipulation. A decision is considered to be free when a person is knowledgeable, has equal access to discussions, and can pursue a course of action without fear of reprisal.

In the "dominance model" of modern medicine, which currently exists, none of these criteria are met [19, pp. 139-141]. Because of their alleged technical skills, physicians are treated as unquestioned authorities. However, other knowledge is involved in treatment that is equally important, which relates to the cultural, social, and moral dimensions of life. In fact, without these background themes, technical issues are practically meaningless. Minus the human presence, technical concerns are vacuous.

Protecting the independence of patients, therefore, requires that the dominance model be dismantled. Dialogic intervention insures this sort of protection. Yet dialogue is anathema to the authority usually accorded to physicians. Dialogue requires reciprocity that many physicians may find unsettling. Nonetheless, dialogue will guarantee that patients are accorded respect. To adopt the language popularized by Buber, an I-thou association is at the core of dialogical interaction, because a "living mutual relation" is enacted between persons [20, p. 19].

Dialogue, according to Habermas, rests on "pure intersubjectivity" [21, p. 143]. What he means is that no *a prioris* should be introduced outside of language to guide discourse. Examples of these extraneous factors are statuses, roles, and traditional claims to power. Interaction can be severely distorted by these considerations, because the strictures they impose are not subject to review. In other words, they do not undergo the interrogation that is part of an unfettered, or purely intersubjective, speech situation.

Due to the reflexive or self-questioning ability of language, a strictly intersubjective interaction has several characteristics that are essential to democratizing the patient-physician relationship. Intersubjective discourse allows for mutual recognition because 1) no norms are exempted from discussion, 2) all claims have a limited range of validity, 3) every assertion is susceptible to critique, and 4) the "I and other" are acknowledged to be competent speakers. As a result, writes Habermas, the ability of persons to express themselves is unimpaired, and thus an unconstrained consensus can be achieved [21, pp. 142-143]. This is a "rational consensus" because the deliberative process is not combative and culminate in forced agreements [22, p. 108]. The prospects for this outcome are enhanced because hidden qualifiers, privileged assumptions, subtle implications, and

traditionally accepted propositions, for example, cannot escape unde-
tected and are vulnerable to critique.

The power of experts depends on their exclusive access to vital
knowledge. This exclusivity is denied by intersubjective discourse.
Although arguments can be made that certain knowledge should be
withheld from the public, for any number of reasons, eventually the
ubiquity of language will prevail. Simply put, language is public; inac-
cessibility to a specific form of knowledge is never complete. To borrow
from Wittgenstein, there is no private language; nothing exceeds the
limits of interpretation and is beyond reproach. Some rules, formulas,
principles, or rights may be designated as "off limits," but this delimita-
tion holds minimal sway as a linguistic form. Nothing that exists
within language, in short, can demand the autonomy coveted by
biomedicine.

With this accessibility to medical knowledge guaranteed, or at least
legitimized, patients can begin to become partners in their treatment.
They can become an "ally in treatment, not the object of it" [5, p. 217].
Specifically important, they can request information that will enable
them to question medical authority and make wise decisions. Once the
uneven distribution of knowledge that prevents dialogue is curtailed,
equalizing the relationship between patient and doctor can begin in
earnest.

BUREAUCRATIC EXCLUSION

At this time, most of the serious policy discussions about health care
are conducted in secret. Sure, public forums are convened, along with
congressional hearings. But practically everyone knows that the real
decisions are not made in these places. Crucial issues and plans,
instead, are addressed by a coterie of persons who are sequestered from
public scrutiny. At the highest echelons of corporate, governmental,
and professional organizations are where the direction of health care
delivery is determined. Accordingly, "all important decisions concerning medical care are entrusted exclusively to professionals who are
responsible only to the medical profession itself or to standards of its
making" [8, p. 98]. The public is thus on the periphery of health care
delivery.

There is no doubt that the purpose of this secrecy is to
protect powerful interests in the medical industry [16, p. 164]. Yet as
might be suspected, another reason is given for these exclusionary
practices. Specifically, efficiency is cited as the rationale for restricting

decision-making. After all, why arouse the ire of the public? If power can be protected without a major confrontation, there is no reason for instigating a political feud. Foucault notes that defusing hostility is possible by making exclusion appear logical [23, p. 140ff.] Instead of angering citizens, they should be convinced that their lack of involvement in health care planning is beneficial. In fact, they have been told that widespread consultations are impractical, inefficient, unwieldy, and too costly.

To reiterate, these are merely excuses for the maintenance of privilege and the guarantee of huge profits. Nonetheless, due to the predominant organizational model, they make sense to the public. In view of the bureaucratization of health care, these reasons for the centralization of decision-making sound prudent [24]. Therefore, the public is cajoled into believing that the best and the brightest persons should be given the sole right to regulate the health care system. This concentration of power, furthermore, is accepted to be entirely legitimate. How else could national decisions be made in a reasonable way?

As argued by Weber, in addition to several newer writers, bureaucracy does not consist simply of a formal linkage between certain roles and statuses [25, pp. 956-1005]. These arrangements represent merely the structural side of bureaucracy. However, this style of organization is underpinned by various beliefs, which comprise a bureaucratic culture or, as Kanter calls it, the "bureaucratic trap" [26, p. 137]. And this constellation of myths has been instrumental in supporting anti-democratic planning in the area of health care.

Although bureaucracies have been tarnished, due to various financial debacles, social research, and attacks by politicians, a number of the themes that are central to these organizations are still popular among the public. First, the hierarchy found in a bureaucracy is thought to be reasonable, because persons have to compete to get to the top. Second, a rigid chain of command is deemed necessary, so as to avoid anarchy and confusion. Third, a fixed system of rules is desirable, for without these directives no one would work. And fourth, consistent with the general theme of science, the formalized and objective logic of a bureaucracy is believed to promote fairness.

What these beliefs have accomplished, nonetheless, is to secure privileged access of a select group of persons to the centers of decision making. As described by Carlson, "Monopolization of authority by bureaucrats led to the creation of an official elite, which in turn discriminated against those less entrenched in the bureaucracy or those outside" [1, p. 129]. Behind a facade of neutrality, the exercise of power goes unchallenged. While most of the public would like to believe that persons with authority deserve to be in these positions, in actuality competition has little to do with promotions. Indeed, the public's fascination with this and the other principles that sustain bureaucracy are unrelated to how this kind of organization functions. Nonetheless, the culture of bureaucracy has become so ingrained that those who criticize these axioms, and sometimes offer alternatives, are dismissed as unrealistic. To the chagrin of many citizens, however, they seem to be regularly betrayed by the organizations they believe are fair and trust.

What has occurred, contends Lefort, is that a totalitarian system has been erected under the guise of objectivity [27, pp. 181-236]. All the while, those with power have been taking advantage of the public's inactivity and good faith. Powerful forces operate behind a cloak of neutrality to fortify their positions, while the general public is hoping to prosper through fair play. This ideology of competence has played a large role in guaranteeing a free rein to those who control organizations. For only persons who are incompetent and unable to compete would dare question the hierarchy that has evolved. The righteousness of privilege thus escapes serious challenge, due to the negative label applied to anyone who is not enamored of status.

Breaking up the clique that conspires to stifle health care reform may have to be achieved through legislation or political force. Either action, however, is no guarantee that the democratization of planning will be the result. Before large-scale participation will become commonplace, the public will have to be convinced that less centralized versions of order are possible. Democratic participation at every level of society, in other words, must not be viewed as some wild utopian vision. Persons must begin to understand that the principles which subtend a bureaucracy are, at best, half-truths. Furthermore, evidence is available which suggests that direct participation in planning results in increased efficiency, improved worker morale, higher output, and, in general, a better attitude toward work than is found in a bureaucracy [26, pp. 129-179]. Instituting "flatter" organizations does not culminate in the disorder that the public has been taught to fear. Just the opposite seems to be true, given the proper preparation. That is, participatory organizations appear to have cultural and social benefits that extend far beyond mere increases in productivity.

There are several models of order that are not based on hierarchy. But the public is told, both overtly and subtly, that these alternatives run counter to everything from human nature to American values.

Nonetheless, order can be preserved through direct discourse that is unmedicated by structural prerequisites, metaphysical props, or myths related to Hobbes' characterization of life. Order does not require the "reality *sui generis*" espoused by social realists, which gradually culminates in bureaucracy. Through learning and effort citizens can become self-directed by acquiring the skill necessary, for example, for them to organize themselves, sensibly allocate resources, and pursue self-imposed goals.

Democracy requires this collective autonomy. Until the public seizes this vision, as opposed to the decrepit one perpetrated by bureaucracy, planning undertaken by exclusive groups will appear sensible. But once true autonomy is appreciated, and the groundwork prepared for its realization, citizens will begin to believe they have the right to confront authority and demand access to formerly private discussions about health care. Contrary to the opponents of democratization, this new social imagery is a fantasy only according to the standards imposed by bureaucracy.

Here, again, dualism must be rejected. The success of non-hierarchial organizations depends on the ability of *praxis* to extend to the core of order. For without the existence of a reality *sui generis*—which preserves the exalted roles, offices, and personal traits essential to hierarchy—the way is clear to initiate a participatory democracy. The distrust of *praxis,* as a viable option to hierarchy, is based on a tradition that understands an absolute reality to be the only workable foundation for order. An organization without structural imperatives, critics claim, would produce a free-for-all, because human action needs direction. Reminiscent of Hobbes, hierarchy is thought to be necessary to control human capriciousness.

This is a bias that has undercut attempts to formulate decentralized conceptions of order, which allow ideas to emerge from every segment of an organization. A directly interactive, or "integral," rendition of organizational life is feasible, once the grip of dualism is released [28, pp. 309-311]. Order emerging from the *vox populi* is not difficult to envision, when dualism is abandoned. In point of fact, democracy is predicated on this notion of participation. Snatching the planning of health care away from experts and other power brokers requires that this non-dualistic social imagery be a part of health care reform. Hence democratic-participatory planning will seem natural, rather than something far fetched.

Nowadays these are referred to as flat or self-managed organizations [29]. With the organization emerging from discourse, institutional

roles are no longer viewed as prescribed or adversarial. These structures, instead, have a pragmatic thrust and reflect collective needs,
rather than natural propensities. Following the change in status of
these strictures, an entrepreneurial spirit can flourish. Nothing
a priori, in short, stands in the way of plans emerging from throughout
an organization.

But as mentioned before, a significant shift in philosophy must
occur prior to this mode of organization coming to be viewed as feasible.
The belief must become prevalent that human, collective action is a
viable source of order. That people can be self-governing must be seen
as a reasonable idea, rather than an invitation to chaos. This realization will only make sense, however, once the search for an absolute
base of order is understood to be interminable and thus foolish. In the
absence of dualism, this search has no justification.

REIFICATION OF GOALS

When discussing health care, everything seems to be ancillary to
economic issues. This obsession is understandable, given that service
delivery is a very profitable business [30, pp. 29-47]. A small change in
one way or another can cost some investors a lot of money. With so
much money hanging in the balance, the importance given to economic
concerns should be of no surprise.

Protecting profit margins, therefore, is a significant part of reform-
ing medicine. Reorganization, accordingly, has assumed the form of
cooperative reorganization, because those who reap the financial
benefits from providing medical care are intent on defining the
parameters of reform [5, p. 77]. As opposed to this method, they could
openly declare their intentions and lose stature in the eyes of their
fellow citizens. For even the most hard-nosed profiteer does not like to
attach a dollar amount to a human life, at least publicly. Therefore, a
less overt strategy had to be devised to insure that certain economic
arrangements are not abridged.

During the 1980s a particular *modus operandi* gained popularity,
although its appearance is not limited to this time period. The aim, in
short, is to make opportunistic definitions—those that serve certain
interests—appear to be natural. The idea is to disperse power by
making particular advantages appear to be "permanent, natural, outside of time" [31, p. 131]. In this way, the exercise of power is legitimized without those who exploit the health care system having to make
crass statements or overtly advocate self-serving policies. As part of the

capitalist system, the market deflects attention away from economic interests.

The market is a shibboleth. Most persons tend to believe that the market is neutral and distributes benefits in a dispassionate manner. By relying on the operation of the market, the average person tends to believe that goods and services will be optimally allocated. The market performs according to laws that are universal, as long as politicians and other meddlers do not upset the precarious balance of forces that is usually maintained. Assessing the potential impact of any change on the market, therefore, is presumed to be economically sound. The centerpiece of rational planning, in short, is market analysis.

A perfect way of maintaining the *status quo* is thus available, without overtly manipulating the public. Simply adhering to the stipulation that the principles of the market, such as free choice, reward for risk, and supply and demand, should not be violated will certainly minimize change. After all, any significant deviation from the present course will be considered an irresponsible challenge to the market. The rules of the market, according to conventional wisdom, do not favor one group over another, but benefit everyone equally. Reality is thus "imploded," as Baudrillard says, without any discernable coercion, for adhering to restrictions imposed by the market does not often alarm anyone [32, pp. 56-57].

By arguing that the market is neutral, intervention is understood to be unneeded. Assumed, however, is that no one controls the market; no one is actively engaged in manipulating this situation. Persons simply compete and await their fate. Given this scenario, there is no reason to believe that the market does not serve everyone equally. Therefore, a *laissez-faire* attitude is engendered among the public, which could prove detrimental to a large segment of the populace.

Specifically, hiding behind the market are vested interests. And these powerful groups, investors, and monopolies are implicitly sanctioned by not contravening the current market conditions. By not piercing the veil of the market, the flow of immense profits to a select few is not seriously threatened. Any plan that would distribute more equitable health care is considered to be antithetical to sound economics. Market relations, as Eagleton writes, are "naturalized and universalized" and made to appear inevitable [33, p. 5]. Domination of the market by a select few is thus surreptitiously legitimized.

Clearly dualism is at the center of this scheme. The existence of natural laws, market forces, and human nature, for example, depends on the ability to sequester these phenomena from situational contingencies. If the market were affected by idiosyncracies, this mechanism would be no more reliable than political events or personal inspiration. The market, however, is supposed to transcend these influences. Yet providing the market with this rarified position gives it the heteronomy necessary to obscure the use of power. Personal gain, at worst, is argued to be an outgrowth of market factors, as opposed to advantage or chicanery. Through dualistic descriptions, the market is elevated above avarice and manipulation.

Viewing the market in this way is not conducive to wide-ranging discussions. Debate is constrained by parameters that are touted to exist *sui generis*. But these qualifications are not thought to be imposed, because they merely reflect the boundaries of economic rationality. No one, in other words, has control over these criteria. At least this is what the public is led to believe.

To avoid this sort of stifling reification, persons must begin to look anew at the economy. Economics does not represent an autonomous realm, but a particular set of priorities. Persons have simply decided to recognize as legitimate certain production relationships, modes of exchange, theories of motivation, and so forth. The claim that workers are motivated by profit, for example, is not necessarily a cultural universal, but a prerequisite of capitalism. Outside of this unique economic system, profit is often insignificant. The commercialization and commodification of relationships is not everyone's ideal.

The point, as raised by Williams, is that economics is a "signifying system" [34, p. 13]. As opposed to an ultimate reality, economics embodies a distinctive manner in which certain values are expressed and reinforced. Economics is merely one way of practicing specific beliefs. Consequently, there is nothing sacrosanct about the prevailing economic imperatives; the currently dominant ideas about economic priorities are not immune to revision.

This is the so-called macro-impact of a dialogical rendition of order. Stated simply, institutionalized goals are not severed from *praxis,* no matter how inviolable they may seem. Grounded in interpretation, the market, and thus all economic strictures, is appreciably affected by shifts in personal or collective interest. Appeals to the market, therefore, do not have the authority of a mandate to stifle change. Instead, the market should reflect shifts in a whole range of priorities, rather than mimic imperatives that are issued by particular economic classes.

From an anti-dualistic perspective, the economy is just another transitory means of revealing human action. Certain themes are instituted, while others are ignored. This particular manifestation of *praxis* is thus fragile, but still capable of having continuity, because there is no cosmology involved in instituting social goals. At best, goals reflect the illusion of permanence, based on the desire to insure their survival, and have "pseudonormative power" [35, pp. 303, 306]. Consistent with the theory of democracy, this anti-dualistic viewpoint allows the current economic priorities to be dismantled and reestablished to meet current needs. Health care can thus reflect the "will of the people," which is the democratic approach for providing institutions with legitimacy.

ESSENTIALISM AND MARGINALIZATION

Seeking a wide range of input is not simply an organizational issue. Health care institutions may become more open, but the number of citizens who participate in debates may remain very small. Again, a particular philosophical viewpoint must be addressed before pluralism and widespread participation are able to come to fruition. This theory results in marginalization, because the assumption is made that worthwhile input originates only from certain groups in the population. Hence the advice or consent of select persons is not often sought. Additionally, information is given little credence when it emanates from these people. As a result of being ignored in this way, large parts of the population may withdraw from civic activities, as apathy becomes pervasive.

Traditionally, a number of persons and groups have been viewed as having little to contribute to public discussions. Blacks and women, for example, have had to fight for minimal recognition. Assumptions were made about their intelligence, ability to reason, and emotional stability that are quite derogatory. Following this degradation, not much effort is expended to integrate fully these persons into the polity. Anything they might have to say, simply put, is thought to be trivial. Said refers to this cultural activity as "a program of ideological pacification" [36, p. 63].

In a society that claims to be democratic, blatant discrimination is outlawed. Therefore, more subtle means of marginalization have been used. One favorite method has been to inferiorize a particular group through what Foucault calls "biopower" [23, p. 140]. This involves substantiating claims about inferiority through recourse to science, physiology, heredity, or other allegedly value-free rationale. Once vital faults are identified, which would definitely require second-class citizenship, persons often readily accept the discriminatory treatment befitting this status. They adjust to what is presumed to be their fate, because the identification of their nature has been undertaken in an allegedly unbiased manner. Through an ostensibly apolitical means, "an atmosphere of submission and of inhibition" is engendered [37, p. 38].

Biopower is predicated on a theory referred to as essentialism [38]. As discussed in Chapter 3, according to this position persons or groups possess an essential core of material or biological "transcendent truths and values" that substantiate fundamental traits [39, p. 221]. The existential dictum is reversed in this case, and essence is understood to precede existence. A person's existence, accordingly, unfolds within predetermined limits that are difficult, if not impossible, to alter. This means that no one is judged to be inferior or superior, but is merely assigned a social role based on intrinsic qualities [40, pp. 109-110]. Values, opinions, or personal feelings have nothing to do with this placement. A teleological explanation is invoked, for example, to justify the disproportionate number of minority persons living below the poverty level. There is no sinister plot, such as class warfare, behind this finding. Ending up in the lower class is simply a matter of destiny, based on a propensity for failure.

With time this outcome may change, as a result of evolution or maturation. But corrective interventions are fruitless, because any marginalization that may occur is a natural occurrence. In fact, implementing remedies through social engineering is considered to be wasteful and, possibly, disruptive. Furthermore, encouraging active participation in social affairs by these marginal persons, through affirmative action, for example, is declared to be dangerous. If these individuals had anything significant to say, according to this argument, they would have been more successful. Seeking their opinions is thus tantamount to fostering the spread of very negative influences, which brought about their undesirable condition in the first place.

Established is an ideology about who is likely to be intelligent, motivated, or hard working. Without the assistance of dualism, however, attaching this type of indelible label to persons would be impossible. For basic to essentialism is the claim that an absolute, or metaphysical, as Sartre writes, identity is present below the surface traits of persons [41, p. 133ff.]. While writing about the inferiorization and murder of Jews, Sartre notes that Hitler's extermination plans were sustained by genetic proof, albeit fictitious, about their decrepit character. Nonetheless, the acceptance of dualism, as reflected in

Descartes' dictum *cogito ergo sum,* allows for this inscrutable and irrefutable justification to be posited.

During a recent program on CNN, for example, the community participation encouraged by the Oregon health plan was symbolically violated. As most persons know by now, citizens were asked to rank treatments in order to prioritize interventions. One expert consultant who was interviewed stated that there appeared to be some "native intelligence" involved in this process [42]. Although this person's intentions may have been honorable, implied is that reason was not operating in establishing this hierarchy of treatments. As opposed to rationality, intuition was at work. Thus a negative image of this proposal was created. Implied was that the population at large should not be involved in this sort of endeavor. This project may have produced sensible results this time, but this outcome was a matter of luck. This is the subtle message conveyed by this CNN broadcast.

But with the demise of dualism, essentialism loses credibility. For this reason, notions such as God and man are outmoded [43]. Accordingly, persons have no other alternative but to invent themselves; there is no essence to justify their existence. Yet recognizing this process reveals the difficulty of identifying persons, *a priori,* according to broad categories. For example, there is no such thing as blacks or women, but different modalities of blackness and femininity. This is not to suggest that certain categories of persons cannot be invented and persecuted. Clearly this has been the case. The point is that even under repressive conditions, personal and group identities are multivalent rather than anchored to a single core. Nothing, even repression, changes the evanescent character of identity and the need to reinvent a self-concept. Moreover, deprived of this absolute referent, advancing claims about inherent inferiority becomes a dubious undertaking. After all, every standard could be subject to debate, even those associated with being superior.

With essentialism under siege, adopting more inclusive practices is relatively easy to do. The new maxim is that input should be judged on its merits, rather than in terms of where this information originated in the social hierarchy. Valuable insight can be found anywhere, once essentialism is jettisoned. Expanding the search for input, therefore, makes good sense and is a sound policy. With a more open vision, new sources of ideas can receive attention, while the thoughts of formerly disenfranchised persons can be seriously reviewed.

In the absence of essentialism, physicians will not be the sole possessors of reason. In fact, reason will be subject to continuous scrutiny and redefinition. For example, biomedical rationality will be understood to represent a particular mode of analysis, which comes to be accepted by a majority of persons. Reason, accordingly, will be viewed to be mixed with political and other forces, which are instrumental in gaining widespread acceptance of a particular viewpoint. As described by Fish, reason will be viewed as a "historical, political, and social product, something that is fashioned by men and women in the name of certain interests, particular concerns, and a social and political agenda" [44, p. 13]. The stage is thus set for privileged symbolism to be questioned—in the form of personal identity or social status—so that true debate can ensue.

CONCLUSION

Various remedies have been proposed throughout the years to cure the crisis in medicine. The thrust of this chapter is to place health care in the current context of attempting to democratize institutions. Implied is that a host of economic or funding proposals may be advanced, but they may not have any real impact until the culture of medicine is democratized.

Democratization is cited to be important for a variety of reasons. On the one hand service delivery can be fine tuned, due to the constant flow of suggestions from citizens. At the same time, efficiency can be improved because of better organizational communication, the elimination of barriers to access, and the closer proximity of services to communities. Democratization, in short, enables services to be directed to concrete individuals and groups, as opposed to the abstractions attendant to the medical model.

Laing makes the case that patients would be helped more by an epistemologist than a physician [45]. His argument is that those who are deemed mad are classified according to an abstract nomenclature, thereby making their behavior seem bizarre. All the while, their actual experiences are systematically occluded. This oversight results in their condition being misunderstood and the prescription of irrelevant services. If a physician should become epistemologically sensitive, on the other hand, this may be the best thing that could happen to a patient.

Such insensitivity is averted by democratization. At the heart of the democratization of medical culture is anti-dualism. Any distance is thus removed from between humans and the institution of medicine. In view of this new closeness, services can be properly focused on patients and their communities. And as a result of this intimacy, the delivery of health care will certainly be improved.

Most important is that democratization is never mentioned in most discussions about formulating a national health care policy. Knowledge bases, organizational styles, and identities, for example, are not linked to opening the health care system. Of course, one could easily say that the present brouhaha is unrelated to opening the medical establishment. Vying for a favorable position at the marketplace is the major preoccupation of those who are debating the future of health care.

Without raising the issue of democratization, however, the delivery of medicine will not change. Even if the public is queried about its preferences, those wishes will not likely be implemented. For the stage has not been set for the advance, recognition, and implementation of divergent ideas. In the absence of critical reflection about the hegemony of biomedicine, medical institutions, and the physician, a more socially responsive system of health care will not be forthcoming. New proposals will be introduced into an ideological framework that will winnow the alternatives until the *status quo* re-emerges. Such an end can be averted only through democratization.

REFERENCES

1. R. J. Carlson, *The End of Medicine,* John Wiley and Sons, New York, 1975.
2. L. Foss and K. Rothenberg, *The Second Medical Revolution: From Biomedicine to Infomedicine,* Shambhala, Boston, 1987.
3. E. Ginzberg, *The Limits of Health Reform,* Basic Books, New York, 1977.
4. M. Haug and B. Lavin, *Consumerism in Medicine: Challenging Physician Authority,* Sage, Beverly Hills, 1983.
5. K. I. Zola, *Socio-Medical Inquiries,* Temple University Press, Philadelphia, 1983.
6. J. S. Maxmen, *The Post-physician Era,* John Wiley and Sons, New York, 1976.
7. C. B. Inlander, L. S. Levin, and E. Weiner, *Medicine on Trial,* Prentice-Hall, New York, 1988.
8. C. C. Havighurst, Why Preserve Private Health Care Financing?, in *American Health Policy: Critical Issues for Reform,* R. B. Helms (eds.), The AEI Press, Washington, D.C., 1993.
9. B. S. Turner, *Medical Power and Social Knowledge,* Sage, Newbury Park, 1987.
10. H. S. Berliner, *A System of Scientific Medicine,* Tavistock, New York, 1985.
11. E. Bittner, The Structure of Psychiatric Influence, *Mental Hygiene, 52*:4, pp. 423-430, 1968.

12. K. Mannheim, The Democratization of Culture, in *From Carl Mannheim,* K. H. Wolff (ed.), Oxford University Press, New York, pp. 271-346, 1971.
13. A. Schutz, *Collected Papers, Vol. I,* Nijhoff, The Hague, 1962.
14. M. Hardt, *Gilles Deleuze: An Apprenticeship in Philosophy,* University of Minnesota Press, Minneapolis, 1993.
15. D. L. Roter and J. A. Hall, *Doctors Talking with Patients / Patients Talking with Doctors,* Aubern House, Westport, Connecticut, 1992.
16. P. Starr, *The Social Transformation of American Medicine,* Basic Books, New York, 1982.
17. J. Habermas, *Autonomy and Solidarity,* Verso, London, 1992.
18. B. Barber, *Informed Consent in Medical Therapy and Research,* Rutgers University Press, New Brunswick, pp. 22-24, 1980.
19. E. Friedson, *Professional Dominance: The Social Structure of Medical Care,* Atherton, New York, 1970.
20. M. Buber, *Between Man and Man,* Macmillan, New York, 1978.
21. J. Habermas, Toward a Theory of Communicative Competence, in *Recent Sociology, No. 2,* H. P. Dreitzol (ed.), Macmillan, New York, 1970.
22. J. Habermas, *Legitimation Crisis,* Beacon Press, Boston, 1973.
23. M. Foucault, *History of Sexuality,* Vol. I, Vintage Books, New York, 1990.
24. D. Mechanic, *Public Expectations and Health Care: Essays on the Changing Organization of Health Services,* Wiley, New York, 1972.
25. M. Weber, *Economy and Society,* Vol. II, University of California Press, Berkeley, 1978.
26. R. M. Kanter, *The Change Masters,* Simon and Schuster, New York, 1984.
27. C. Lefort, *The Political Forms of Modern Society,* MIT Press, Cambridge, Massachusetts, 1986.
28. J. Gebser, *The Ever-present Origin,* Ohio University Press, Athens, Ohio, 1985.
29. J. W. Murphy, Organizational Issues in Worker Ownership, *The American Journal of Economics and Sociology, 43,* pp. 287-299. 1984.
30. D. Mechanic, *From Advocacy to Allocation: The Evolving American Health Care System,* The Free Press, New York, 1986.
31. J. B. Thompson, *Studies in the Theory of Ideology,* University of California Press, Berkeley, 1984.
32. J. Baudrillard, *Simulations,* Semiotext(e), New York, 1983.
33. T. Eagleton, *Ideology,* Verso, London, 1991.
34. R. Williams, *Culture,* Fontana, London, 1989.
35. J. Habermas, *Knowledge and Human Interests,* Beacon Press, Boston, 1971.
36. E. Said, Interview, *Z Magazine,* July/August 1993.
37. F. Fanon, *The Wretched of the Earth,* Grove Weidenfield, New York, 1991.
38. S. Bordo, Feminism, Postmodernism, and Gender-Skepticism, in *Feminism / Postmodernism,* J. Nicholson (ed.), Routledge, New York, pp. 133-156, 1990.

39. S. Fish, *Doing What Comes Naturally,* Duke University Press, Durham, 1989.
40. U. Gerhardt, *Ideas About Illness,* New York University Press, New York, 1989.
41. J.-P. Sartre, *Anti-Semite and Jew,* Schocken, New York, 1969.
42. *News from Medicine,* Cable News Network, August 31, 1992.
43. M. Foucault, *The Order of Things,* Tavistock, London, 1970.
44. S. Fish, Canon Busting: The Basic Issues, *National Forum, 69,* 1989.
45. R. D. Laing, The Mystification of Experience, in *Radical Psychology,* P. Brown (ed.), Harper and Row, New York, pp. 109-127, 1973.

CHAPTER
8

Conclusion

Clearly, a new dimension must be added to the current debate about national health care. Due to the focus on the market, and the accompanying realism, concerns have been raised thus far about patients having the free choice of doctors, government involvement in the creation of a medical bureaucracy, the affordability of any plan, the impact of a national program on doctors, insurance companies, and pharmaceutical firms, and the increase in the current budget deficit that may be necessary to finance any reforms. As might be expected, conspicuously absent in all of this discussion is any mention of democratization. Every other institution is believed to benefit from an infusion of democracy, so why not the medical system?

Although the President was coy about this issue, special interests did keep trying to sway Hillary Rodham Clinton and the committee she chaired. The general public has received only bits and pieces of information, while powerful lobbyists have been bombarding Mrs. Clinton's committee with a myriad of so-called "bottom line" threats. If a policy is adopted that is antagonistic to their interests, these mysterious characters exclaim, the President will lose their support and his health care initiative will collapse. Behind the scenes, these individuals are attempting to squander the health of the American public. Nothing seems to matter but their personal gain.

The medical system could easily qualify as totalitarian [1, p. 89]. Isolated from the general public, the medical establishment is insulated from most criticism. Outside of litigation, which the average citizen cannot afford and does not understand, persons have little to say about how they are treated. And once they are inside of the system, patients are swept along by faceless experts until the money runs out or treatment is terminated [2]. Patients are willingly provided with a minimal amount of information, processed, and discharged. All the time, their health is in the hands of a medical team they have no ability to control. What could be more Kafkaesque?

In order to maintain this system, health care has become a commodity that fewer and fewer persons can buy. In a word, privilege, power, and profits must be preserved. As a result, the system tightens; the wagons are circled for protection. Attention is directed away from practically everything but cost. Regardless of what is proposed, free enterprise must not be jeopardized. And to the benefit of those on Wall Street and certain medical professionals, medical costs continue to rise. At the same time, the "spin doctors" hired by the AMA and drug companies are busy scaring the public into believing that its "freedom to choose" is about to be usurped. The loser in the end is the citizenry, who are left to face a medical monolith that escapes unscathed.

Like most undemocratic regimes, the present medical system is corrupt and inefficient. Without outside monitors and a forum for public discussion, inside deals are regularly made that enhance the medical establishment, but are detrimental to the public. Furthermore, services are offered that are irrelevant, inappropriate, and, sometimes, damaging [3, pp. 21-44]. All the while the meter is running. And when something goes wrong, everyone denies responsibility or knowledge, or doctors claim they are only human, and the only recourse remaining for patients is litigation or silent suffering.

If democracy had been operative, however, this sort of adversary relationship could have been avoided. Doctors and patients could collaborate, and thereby begin to share responsibility for a course of action. Likewise, research could be a joint endeavor, so that the newest findings could be disseminated rapidly throughout society. The point is that thoroughly informed decisions could be made by everyone involved, and thus no one will feel slighted by the outcome of an intervention. As Lewin demonstrated, everyone will be "bought into" the entire treatment process [4]. In the end, suspicion and resistance can be replaced by cooperation, so that timely, efficient, and effective health care can be provided.

The idea is not simply that all parties must communicate. Without the dismantling of power and other impediments to participation, true dialogue is impossible. As discussed in Chapter 7, certain conditions must be met before citizens can become thoroughly involved in their treatment. A type of symmetry must be present between all the persons involved. Unless this is the case, communication will take the form of imperatives or ultimatums issued by those who hold key social positions. Although communication is a vital part of democracy, other factors must be in place before real discussion occurs.

GIVING DEMOCRACY A CHANCE

Key to democratization is that institutions are a collective undertaking or, as Englehardt states, the result of a "communal decision" [5, p. 196]. The "will of the people" is considered to be central to social life, so that the polity reflects "participation on a daily basis by the working classes and popular masses in all economic, political, and social institutions" [6, p. 177]. Immersing medicine in the daily affairs of citizens, accordingly, is required by democratization. Connecting the delivery of health care to the people is the aim of this process.

As discussed earlier, society cannot be democratized in the absence of a culture of democracy. This finding is also true for medicine. One way to inaugurate democratization is to pursue some themes that are vital to opening the institution of medicine. The following are some important points for discussion that are germane to making health care less autonomous and more socially responsible. But due to the focus directed to cost accounting, these ideas have been overshadowed.

Attacking medicine is not enough to insure that democratization will occur. Demanding openness is only one step toward requiring institutions to reflect the will of the people. A proper outlook, culture or spirit, is necessary to support institutional changes that lead to democracy. Raising certain key points can serve as a segue to this end.

HEALTH CARE AS A COMMODITY VERSUS A RIGHT

For example, at this time health care is treated mostly as a commodity. Medical interventions, in short, are generally available to those who can purchase them. Having the proper skills, job, family background, and so forth are the requisites for receiving treatment. But when persons do not even have the right to work, as a fundamental human activity, medical care will never be delivered in more than a haphazard way.

When health care is understood to be a basic right, there is no reason why universal medical coverage that is acceptable is impossible to provide. Indeed, special interests threatening to drop out of the planning process would be considered unconscionable and worthy of prosecution. And squabbles over the cost of a package would be ancillary to providing the services. Clearly, many authorities are searching for these and other excuses for not offering universal health care. A wise step would be to acknowledge that adequate health care is a basic right, something essential to securing "species-typical functioning" and operate within this context [7, pp. 26-28]. Light could thus be shed on what is meant by a society having the obligation to supply all citizens with health care.

INFORMED CITIZENS

Democracy is impossible unless persons have the information necessary for institutions to function effectively. Most persons have little understanding of health promotion, diagnosis, the use of medicine, or treatment options. In many cases serious problems could be avoided, with a minimal preventive effort or knowledge of a few simple interventions. Left in the dark, however, citizens cannot participate meaningfully in the health care system.

In order to create a health conscious society—as opposed to one that is obsessed with heroic, grandiose, and highly technical correctives—a full discussion of health and health promotion should be inaugurated. In this regard, ways of disseminating information, gathering the most diverse input, developing forums for public discussions, and monitoring the delivery of services should be explored. As a result, a fully informed citizenry can be promoted, thereby enabling these persons to take control of the medical institution. With the application of medicine demythologized, the entire health care system can be made socially responsive. And because of this improved supervision, service delivery will likely improve.

Many state health plans are currently under review that have been inaugurated with "public hearings," the formation of "advisory committees," "task forces," and "town meetings." The aim of this process, of course, is to allow for local input, which would be consistent with democracy [8]. Nonetheless, as Carlson argues, the "idea of community implies increased local control" [9, p. 149]. His point is that allowing uninformed citizens to talk does not provide their sentiments with credibility. Moreover, their presence represents merely tokenism if they are placed in a situation which those in power control and are unwilling to change. For example, often these task forces are comprised of persons who have little or no relationship to the communities in question, and in fact define the parameters of discussion.

RELEVANT SERVICES

Another area that needs attention relates to the delivery of pertinent services. At this juncture, interventions seem to be more service than patient oriented. An array of services is developed mostly in terms of professional expertise, available technology and facilities, and cost. Within these boundaries, patients are given a choice of treatments. The problem is that a patient's needs may fit only marginally into the resulting network of services. Luck more than anything else may determine whether services are provided in a culturally sensitive and technically competent manner.

A serious discussion is needed, accordingly, about how to identify problems and supply services that are socially relevant. Both theory and technique should be given serious attention. With regard to the former, a new theory of service organization, philosophy of science, rationale for making a diagnosis, and research methodology must be formulated. On the other hand, alternative approaches to locating service agencies, identifying access points, and aligning services with a community's cultures, values, and priorities must be elevated in importance. In this way, the practice of medicine can become truly integrated into a community, thus fostering the efficient use of services.

For example, the methodology of the Oregon Plan has been criticized for being socially insensitive. Cost seemed to be the focus of attention, in the form of cost-utility analysis, while the characteristics of a community were never made clear. Some groups were excluded, while those who attended town meetings did not represent the community as a whole. In the end, claims La Puma, "community preferences [were] based on hypothetical medical situations over the preferences of individual patients" [10, p. 128]. To avoid this difficulty, both theory and methods must be devised that are not merely objective, but are sensitive to the life-world of a community. The focus should not be on data, but on context-based information. Accordingly, new, more interpretive methodologies that are socially sensitive must be invented. Entrée to communities must be gained, so that proper services are provided in the most appropriate manner. Otherwise, health care will be supplied haphazardly.

A PUBLIC SYSTEM

Many critics charge that there is no health care system in the United States. The argument is that treatment is available for only a portion of the population, and that even these services do not constitute an integrated system. Contrary to this view, there appears to be a myriad of systems, which sometimes conflict with one another. A maze of services exist that is disorganized, compartmentalized, defies regulation, and, in general, swallows patients upon entry. Due to this lack of organization, well known, generally available, and universal services, which are characteristics usually adopted to define "public," are rare. The waste that results from such fragmentation is astronomical.

What needs to be addressed is the concept of public services. Specifically noteworthy, in this regard, is what is meant by the term "public" in the context of medicine? Does this mean that patients should have direct access to a holistic system of community-based clinics? Or does this term mean that the present public facilities—schools, libraries, and community centers, for example—should be organized into a comprehensive system of primary prevention and intervention? In the past, public health has pertained to the social side of medicine, including education, nutrition, and sanitation, for example. Within the framework of democratization, however, the meaning of "the public" must be expanded to encompass issues related to community support of services, patient advocacy, control of agencies, review of research, and the direct involvement of the public in funding decisions. If the medical institution is going to be public, this idea must be clarified and a compatible service system designed.

EDUCATING HEALERS

The type of education physicians typically receive should be rethought. Although medical students are intimately tied to the public—through grants, loans, and other means of support for study—they tend to view themselves as "free agents." They begin to conduct themselves as merchants who sell their technical wares to the highest bidder. They tend to engage in what Zola calls "entrepreneurial practice," which may only be indirectly related to meeting the needs of the public [11, p. 78]. Although they are supported for years by public largess, many physicians are socialized to believe they are self-made persons who have the right to pursue any career path they desire. But any sense of reciprocity would dictate that such an attitude or behavior is unfair.

As opposed to merchants, physicians should begin to view themselves as healers [12, pp. 92-129]. Traditionally, healers have held a special role in communities. They have been granted a unique status, due to their intimate knowledge of a community's heritage, customs, *raison d'être,* and needs. In short, a healer has an inviolable responsibility toward a community whereas a merchant does not [13, p. 114]. In more modern parlance, physicians should receive more of a service orientation. Perhaps like social workers, members of the medical team should be taught they have an almost sacred obligation to promote the common weal, above all else. What needs to be addressed is the details of how this attitude can be incorporated into the core of medical education.

COLLECTIVE RESOURCE ALLOCATION

Given their love affair with capitalism, Americans have a fascination with the market. The cost of goods and services, stated simply, is thought to be arrived at through free exchange at the market place. But medical costs have continued to rise, even though the public is generally disgruntled about the way in which services are delivered. The rationale for this market anomaly is quite simple. Persons are reluctant to negotiate price when they are sick or facing a medical emergency. And given the current monopoly that exists with regard to services, the market can hardly be expected to function effectively [14, pp. 25-26].

If the market is going to work in this area, citizens and representatives of the health care system must be able to negotiate the cost of services in a non-emergency or non-coercive setting. Persons should be able to assess collectively how much of their resources they are willing to devote to medical care. In almost all of the discussions in which citizens have been included, this sort of option has not existed [1, p. 310]. Nonetheless, a sort of national health budget could be established, with persons having the opportunity to discuss the percentage of their household income that they think should be allocated to medical care.

Daniels refers to this activity as "explicit, democratically accountable rationing," whereby services are allocated according to a "public process according to resource limitations" [15, p. 189]. Parameters could thus be set for determining a fair price, which are divorced from entrenched institutions, power, and predetermined views about health, which everyone is expected to respect [16, p. 226]. Consistent with democracy, these constraints will be self-imposed and have enhanced legitimacy, if they truly reflect the will of the community. Working out the details of this citizen-wide mode of collective bargaining will be very challenging, but is vital to allowing the market to allocate health care.

This national budget, however, is different in several ways from what some writers are calling a "global budget" [17]. To insure cost containment, the idea is now circulating among policy makers that a cap should be placed on spending for health care. But this global budget does not necessarily embody a spirit of democracy. Vested economic interests, so-called structural aspects of the economy, or expectations about returns on investments, for example, are not necessarily questioned. A truly national health care budget, on the other hand, is not constructed from within traditional economic laws or expectations. Rather, nothing is excluded from negotiation and a budget emerges that reflects the preferences that are critically examined during this process.

THE WILL OF THE PEOPLE

When institutions are thought to emerge from the "will of the people," many commonly tolerated conditions will be viewed differently. For example, institutions will not be viewed as "out of control," change will be understood as unrestricted, rules and laws will not be viewed as intractable, policy "realities" will not be treated as imperatives, and authorities will not be autonomous. In a democracy the people give legitimacy to institutions, and through serious deliberation they have the ability to recall officials or revise policies. Considering these traits, medicine would be affected drastically by democracy becoming an integral part of the health care system.

When institutions become antagonistic to social interests, and begin to erode persons' confidence and future, something has gone drastically wrong. Persons have become thoroughly alienated and, as a result, self-destructive. They have forgotten, in other words, that they support institutions, rather than the other way around, and are dominated, intimidated, and, in the end, controlled by their creations.

While the concept of "peoples participation" in health care has been utilized mostly in the third world, this idea is integral to democracy [18, p. 23]. Persons serve as agents of change, who eliminate any traditional barriers to the optimal use of medical services, including systems of inequalities. Patients make informed decisions about needs, identify acceptable remedies, supervise the delivery of services, and evaluate outcomes. Most important, however, is that medicine is fit into the image persons have of their existence. Medicine is simply one facet of persons creating and maintaining their lives, which has no predetermined limits.

Those who are invested in protecting the *status quo* in health care will fight the institution of democracy. The reason why is that nothing should escape discussion and critique; there is no "bottom line" that must be adopted. Reality is no longer reified, as when apologies are offered for the prevailing social arrangements. The aim of democracy is to allow persons to become self-reliant, rather than enslaved to predetermined ideas or practices. In the case of health care, persons will be allowed to take control of their well-being.

Although more services and dollars should be devoted to medical care, research suggests that increases in these areas alone are insufficient to improve the health of a population [18, pp. 37-39]. More significant is that the impediments to effective utilization be eliminated. Often the social conditions that created medical problems are left untouched, even though services have been expanded. As suggested earlier, the basis of democracy is the removal of factors that do not reflect human *praxis*. After all, advocates of democracy ask, why would persons repress themselves through the enactment of oppressive policies? Indeed, when alienation is replaced by self-sufficiency, institutions are thought to chart a path of self-actualization rather than control persons. With the institution of democracy, accordingly, allowing medicine to remain antagonistic to the human condition makes no sense.

NEITHER MARKET NOR STATE

Usually talk about health care has two foci, either the market or the state. In the case of the market, consumer sovereignty is considered to be most important. Customers, in short, are free to pursue their own aims, and as a result exert pressure on businesses to provide relevant and high quality goods and services. Yet in actuality, consumers are often uninformed, disorganized, and easily manipulated. They do not act rationally, as assumed by exponents of the market, and regularly contravene their own interests. They are atoms that act frenetically.

The state, on the other hand, is no better informed. Interference from the state is supposed to counter the influence of powerful forces, so that the average citizen is not overrun. Nonetheless, state officials have become an impenetrable clique, which is far removed from the citizenry and unduly indebted to those with power. In the classic sense of bureaucracy, the state does not reasonably distribute resources, but consumes them in ever increasing amounts. The state has become the faceless adversary of most persons.

In the case of health care, neither of these approaches has proven to be workable. The medical cartel has subverted a true market situation. Relying on the market, therefore, in its current monopolistic condition, has simply allowed powerful interests to take advantage of an unmonitored situation. Waste and fraud, however, are usually a part of allowing the state to operate institutions, such as hospitals. As a result, a third road must be tried, one that is often talked about but seldom adopted. Stated succinctly, the people should be allowed to truly govern themselves.

"Grass roots" politics should be taken seriously. Usually, however, this style of political action is considered to be anachronistic, or possibly frivolous. As a result, the political pundits stress everything but the right of persons to invent the polity and guide its growth. Parties, political action committees, and lobbyists, for example, are treated as influential, while the actual centerpiece of democracy is overlooked. With regard to recent developments in medicine, specifically in the example of Oregon, the Health Services Commission intervened and revised the list of interventions, when the ranking of services did not make sense to the experts. Democracy was thus contravened. Still, in a democratic polity, power originates from the grass roots, contrary to the way in which this notion is often portrayed. Rather than a quaint idea, grass roots politics is the heart and soul of democracy. Should citizens become angry enough, power that is not supported at this level can be extinguished.

As suggested by Habermas with his notion of the ideal speech situation, vital to a grass roots orientation is that every agenda starts from a zero base. Every proposal is debated in an environment free of coercion, manipulation, intimidation, and interest groups, because of their size and influence, that can dictate the range of discussion. Both the market and state, on the other hand, do not necessarily challenge traditional social arrangements in their attempt to regulate society. Their respective methods of allocation regularly begin *in medias res,* or take for granted the legitimacy of the present order.

Grass roots politics, to borrow from Marx, is much more radical. Every institution, in short, is examined against the backdrop of political will, or the zero base of the polity. Nothing is sacrosanct, except the ability of the people to select and embark on a course of action. These options are debated and prioritized, with steps taken to insure that minorities receive equal representation. Further, care is taken to insure that rankings can be rotated with ease. No prevailing tradition or institution, in other words, has the latitude to block the will of the citizenry.

Any serious attempt to democratize medicine requires that this institution be built from the "ground up." Through discussion at the lowest level, possibly the neighborhood, a working consensus can be developed about the future of health care. At the minimum, a slate of proposals can be developed for a general discussion. The point is that those who are really intent on changing medicine must address how input from the grass roots can be tapped.

Most important is that this input is not simply opinion. Real democracy does not rest on a bifurcation between opinion and reality. In other words, there is no reason for separating political will from institutions, and thereby erect the conditions that would inhibit *praxis*. Portraying the polity in this dualistic manner would merely undermine initiative, because human action would be confronted constantly by institutions that have an objective status. Desires would be met regularly head-on by an unrelenting reality.

In concrete terms, once this seignorial reality is recognized to be something special, those who have power can easily use it to their advantage. Through propaganda and other means of manipulation, this option can come to be viewed as natural, normative, and thus inviolable. Medical officials have often used this strategy to convince citizens that any substantial change would dismantle the best system of care that has ever existed. From a grass roots viewpoint, however, input is not deflected by reality, but instead reaches to the core of the polity. As Lefort argues, following the collapse of dualism, reality constitutes a "social imaginary" that is insubstantial [19, pp. 200-201]. In this sense, political action is understood to invent and sustain the polity. Citizens are thus free to give legitimacy to any number of realities; they are able to "freely associate" in a variety of ways. Consequently, they are less susceptible to threats about impending doom, if a traditional institution is challenged.

The "rationality of the real" is found nowhere else but in discourse. Divorced from discourse, "managed competition" and a "single player," for example, may have little to do with insuring equity, relevance, or the effectiveness of health care. Competition that is not based on discourse can easily become nothing more than conglomerates vying for power, which does not preclude mergers, price fixing, joint planning, and other measures that perpetuate market advantages. But once primacy is given to discourse, *a prioris* dissolve and all outcomes are predicated on human agency. In this way institutions and their administration are truly public. Rather than assumed, societal arrangements are within the public domain and open to criticism [20, pp. 182-183]. There are no guarantees, accordingly, about the course or outcome of dialogue.

THE OREGON SYSTEM: DEMOCRACY IN ACTION?

During the late 1980s, Oregon faced many budgetary problems similar to other states. Particularly relevant to this discussion is that the costs of the Medicaid program, a federal and state jointly-funded program to provide health care for the poor, had been growing at an annual rate of 25 percent [21, p. 154]. Without enormous increases in revenue, Medicaid services would have to be curtailed soon. As the citizens of Oregon saw the problem, funding may have to be stopped for expensive and highly risky procedures, such as organ transplants, so that more basic practices could be extended throughout the low-income population. Medicaid, in short, had to be rationed. But the easy way out, taken by many states, is to change eligibility criteria and exclude certain persons from treatment. The citizens of Oregon chose the more difficult path, and decided overtly to ration services.

On the basis of forty-eight town meetings and twelve public hearings, which were attended by approximately one-thousand persons, a set of community values emerged. Prevention, for example, was argued to be more important than expensive heroic interventions that benefit only a small number of persons. But in order to focus on prevention, spending had to be reduced in other areas. Therefore, citizens were also asked to prioritize interventions—through a telephone survey of 1001 respondents—with regard to cost, net benefit, and social importance. A treatment that was costly and had limited impact, both in terms of its usage rate and effectiveness, was viewed as less important than one that is inexpensive, widely used, and very effective.

In the end, a list of 709 paired conditions and treatments was generated, and funds were allocated by the state legislature to fund services down to number 587. Indeed, this ranking was used to guide budgetary decisions during the 1991 legislative session. Hence 98 percent of the services classified as "essential to basic care" were funded, along with 82 percent of the services referred to as "very important" and 7 percent of those categorized as "valuable to individuals but of normal gain and/or high cost" [22, p. 39].

Because of this participatory process, the Oregon plan is thought to be a move in the right direction toward democratic medicine. As described by Engelhardt:

> Oregon's approach to health care involves the straightforward recognition that citizens must consider how much of their common resources they wish to set aside for health care for the poor, and which health care goods and services they wish to purchase [5, p. 203].

While the outcome of this process may not be ideal, he goes on to state that "Oregon represents the first substantial attempt to democratize discussions regarding health care allocations" [5, p. 204]. The purpose of health care was debated in public, and the citizenry proposed a method of organizing services that reflects its desires. In this regard, Englehardt is correct that Oregon has done better than other states and the federal government in allowing persons, through a collective process, to establish an agenda for health care services.

Despite this praise, there are some shortcomings of the process used by Oregonians that should not be overlooked. These defects relate to two areas: technical issues pertaining to the methodology adopted to generate the list of treatments, and problems that jeopardized the democratic nature of the undertaking. Due to the thrust of this book, the second point will be addressed.

First, this process was inaugurated within strict economic guidelines. Rationing, simply put, could not violate the already existing Medicaid budget. But other alternatives are available, ranging from a Canadian-style plan to other models found in Europe. Higher taxes could have been levied, or health care could have been viewed as a benefit all those who contribute to society should receive. The citizens of Oregon, therefore, did not really have a free and open discussion, because the health care options were specified prior to the onset of debate. What they had, according to Paul Feyerabend, was a "guided exchange," whereby discussion took place within predetermined parameters [23, pp. 29-30]. Thus the validity of proposals did not emerge from discussion; the boundaries of discussion did not evolve from dialogue.

Second, the knowledge necessary to make informed decisions about the efficacy of treatments was not disseminated throughout the population [21, p. 152]. There seemed to be a bias from the start that ordinary citizens could not really accomplish this task. As a result, complaints began to emerge shortly after the list was published, which suggested that the priorities adopted by citizens were not rational. Some traditional standards of medicine, in short, were abridged, thus calling into question this method of distributing health care. Experts believed the reasoning of citizens was somehow faulty and called into question the entire undertaking. Aspersions were thus cast on popular control of medicine. The will of the people, in short, was inferiorized by biomedicine.

Third, in the end experts dominated the process of allocating services. When the list appeared to be counterintuitive to medical officials, the Health Service commissioners intervened and made what they believed to be the necessary corrections. Note should be taken that more than half of these individuals were health care professionals. And as argued by Daniels, spurning the community in this way means that the rankings are "really the result of an indirect democratic process, and not a participatory one" [15, p. 191]. In effect, when the community deviated from the opinion of experts, discussion ended. Clearly this is paternalism and should not be a part of democracy.

Fourth, standard practices were used to gain citizen input, without establishing the conditions required for widespread discussions. As a result, the charge has been raised that attendance at the town meetings was poor and insufficient to justify policy changes [10, p. 128]. Phone surveys and community meetings are typical strategies, which may be ineffective if persons are not used to participatory government. Before public forums are initiated, a cultural framework must be developed that encourages participation and insures the direct flow of input into the planning process. Furthermore, actual schemes should be formulated that make widespread participation easy and complete.

And fifth, only one aspect of the Oregon health care system was considered to be problematic and revamped. That is, the primary concern is that providing medical services to the poor is too costly. Of course this group of persons was only marginally involved in the public meetings. Perhaps more serious is that this group was isolated and not viewed to be part of a larger public, which is an attitude that perpetuates the problems of the poor. Implied is that only certain aspects of the policy are accessible for discussion, while other domains are sacrosanct. Specifically, the rich can do as they please, while the poor are left to fight among themselves for minimal services. Questioning the social nature of wealth is deemed irresponsible; a minimal standard of living for everyone is utopia. Anselm Strauss is correct when he says that equal health care will not come about until the entire medical system is revised [24, p. 71]. Tinkering with merely one segment of a defective system will not appreciably improve health care [22, p. 54].

A PARTICIPATORY ENVIRONMENT

A key finding of the 1980s is that ideas have power. The market, and all its imagery, became a vital component of the American psyche. In terms of democracy the message is clear: ideas that are compatible with this mode of politics must be developed and widely disseminated. Like the market, these images of democracy must become almost second nature.

For example, persons must begin to recognize that they are essentially connected, rather than atoms, and exist in solidarity with others [5, p. 196]. They must begin to understand that they are not part of a government, but are self-governing. Rather than using institutions, they invent them. The aim is not simply to convince persons that they are free—which has come to mean free to accept or make changes at the margins of the prevailing reality—but to empower them [25, p. 7]. The end product is supposed to be citizens who will accept nothing less than full participation in society.

At the same time, mechanisms for this participation must be formulated. For as Daniels writes, the "primary obligations in the distribution of health care are social rather than the individual or professional obligations of the physician" [7, pp. 116-117]. Priority should thus be given to organizing communities, so that information can be accumulated and disseminated. Community-based monitoring of the resulting institutions is important, along with rules for making changes once a particular course of action is selected. As might be suspected, not much information exists about planning participatory health care organizations. This endeavor has been turned over to medical experts, allied health professionals, and those companies and interests that comprise the health care industry. A people-supported, or thoroughly democratic, health care system would be something new.

In the end, though, only a democratic health care system will meet the needs of the people. Without any intermediaries, they will collectively allocate resources to health care. Moreover, they will be involved directly in determining whether their needs have been met. Some critics might say this proposal is idealistic. But what could be more realistic than persons having a clear understanding of the resources that are available, their optimal distribution and use, and the most relevant measures of evaluation? The key difference with the past is that citizens would have this information, instead of only the medical establishment. In an allegedly democratic society, this idea should not sound so foreign or impossible.

This is not to say, however, that a shift in philosophy is sufficient to alter the present medical system. On this count Fish is correct [26, pp. 431-432]. That is, the critical insight spawned by reflexive theory is not enough to bring about a full-fledged cultural revolution. Shifts in consciousness, simply put, do not necessarily translate into political upheavals. There is no doubt that political muscle will be required to produce an all-inclusive health care policy. But the acquisition and exercise of power without the insight provided by reflexivity can be disastrous. Another autonomous seat of power, similar to the one occupied by biomedicine, may be instituted. If this were to happen, nothing would be achieved by a revolution. To paraphrase Marx, theory is the mind of change, while politics is the heart of any movement.

Up until this juncture both of these components have been wrong. The point of this book is to show how several theoretical currents combined to produce a particular practice of medicine, which has declining utility and a huge price tag. Rectifying this situation will require a general theoretical reorientation, along with a technically mature body politic.

But most of the public debates thus far have been devoid of this sort of theorizing. Accordingly, the authors of this text have provided a glimpse at an emerging paradigm, in addition to its political side. And in view of the call that is made to democratize medicine, providing this information is especially challenging. That is, themes that are vital to democracy are addressed, but without detailing how this style of medicine should be achieved. Such prescriptions would be counter-productive. The implementation must come from the people. Clearly, democratization has promise for providing what most citizens want—a responsive system of health care. Creating this approach to medicine, however, demands that a host of firmly entrenched themes be rethought. Therefore, good theory will be available to guide appropriate practice. Contrary to some popular opinions, theory is connected to reality. And illustrating this relationship is at the core of this book.

REFERENCES

1. C. C. Havighurst, Why Preserve Private Health Care Financing?, in *American Health Policy: Critical Issues for Reform*, R. B. Helms (ed.), AEI Press, Washington, D.C., 1993.

2. E. Goffman, *Asylums,* Doubleday, New York, 1961.
3. I. Illich, *Limits to Medicine,* Penguin Books, New York, 1977.
4. K. Lewin, Frontiers in Group Dynamics, *Human Relations, Vol. 1,* pp. 5-47, 1947.
5. H. T. Englehardt, Jr., Why a Two-Tier System of Health Care is Morally Unavoidable, in *Rationing America's Medical Care: The Oregon Plan and Beyond,* M. A. Strosberg, J. M. Wiener, R. Baker, and I. A. Fine (eds.), The Brookings Institution, Washington, D.C., 1992.
6. V. Navarro, *Crisis, Health, and Medicine,* Tavistock, New York, 1986.
7. N. Daniels, *Just Health Care,* Cambridge University Press, Cambridge, 1985.
8. *State Initiatives in Health Care Reform, No. 3,* The Alpha Center, Washington, D.C., 1993.
9. R. J. Carlson, *The End of Medicine,* John Wiley and Sons, New York, 1975.
10. J. LaPuma, Quality-Adjusted Years: Why Physicians Should Reject the Oregon Plan, in *Rationing America's Health Care: The Oregon Plan and Beyond,* M. A. Strosberg, I. M. Wiener, R. Baker, and I. A. Fine (eds.), The Brookings Institution, Washington, D.C., 1992.
11. K. I. Zola, *Socio-medical Inquiries,* Temple University Press, Philadelphia, 1975.
12. R. M. Zaner, *Ethics in the Clinical Encounter,* Prentice-Hall, Englewood Cliffs, New Jersey, 1988.
13. M. Johnson, *Moral Imagination,* University of Chicago Press, Chicago, 1993.
14. T. R. Marmor, The Right to Health Care: Reflections on its History and Politics, in *Rights to Health Care,* T. J. Bole, III, and W. B. Bondeson (eds.), Kluwer, Dordrecht, 1991.
15. N. Daniels, Justice and Health Care Rationing: Lessons from Oregon, in *Rationing America's Health Care: The Oregon Plan and Beyond,* M. A. Strosberg, J. M. Wiener, R. Baker, and I. A. Fine (eds.), The Brookings Institution, Washington, D.C., 1992.
16. N. K. Rhoden, Free Markets, Consumer Choice, and the Poor: Some Reasons for Caution, in *Rights to Health Care,* T. J. Bole, III and W. B. Bondeson (eds.), Kluwer, Dordrecht, 1991.
17. S. Altman and A. B. Cohen, The Need for a National Global Budget, *Health Affairs, 12,* pp. 194-203, 1993.
18. S. B. Rifkin, *Health Planning and Community Participation,* Croom Helm, London, 1985.
19. C. Lefort, *The Political Forms of Modern Society,* MIT Press, Cambridge, Massachusetts, 1986.
20. J. Habermas, *Autonomy and Solidarity,* Verso, London, 1992.
21. R. M. Kaplan, *The Hippocratic Predicament,* Academic Press, San Diego, 1993.

22. M. J. Garland, Rationing in Public: Oregon's Priority-setting Methodology, in *Rationing America's Medical Care: The Oregon Plan and Beyond,* M. A. Strosberg, J. M. Wiener, R. Baker, and I. A. Fine (eds.), The Brookings Institution, Washington, D.C., 1992.
23. P. Feyerabend, *Science in a Free Society,* NLB, London, 1978.
24. A. L. Strauss, Medical Ghettos, in *Where Medicine Fails,* A. L. Strauss (ed.), Transaction Books, New Brunswick, New Jersey, 1984.
25. H. Marcuse, *One-dimensional Man,* Beacon Press, Boston, 1964.
26. S. Fish, *Doing What Comes Naturally,* Duke University Press, Durham, 1989.

Index

Aging: and appropriate treatment, 90-91; and biomedicine, 83, 84, 85; and chronic disease, 83-89; and diet, 89-90; and environmental medicine, 87-88; and the failure of biomedicine, 91-92; and health maintenance, 87-88; increasing incidence of, 86-89; and medicare, 84-85; and long-term care, 83-84, 90

Andral, G., 65

Auenbrugger, L., percussion, 58

Arney, W., 57

Bacon, R., 60

Barber, G., 45

Barthes, R., language use, 101; the life-world (*Lebenswelt*), 114; photography, 59; physiology, 18-19; the self, 103

Basch, S. von, 63

Baudrillard, J., implosion of reality, 135

Becker, H., moral entrepreneurs, 112

Behavioral medicine, description of, 77-78

Bergen, B., 57

Berliner, H., 124

Bichat, X., 55, 57, 61, 62

Binswanger, L., being-in-the-world, 104

Biomedical model: and aging, 82-89, 91; and the alienation of patients, 122-123; and causality, 22-24, 43, 107-108, 110; and chronicity, 89; components of, 1-2, 33, 48-49; and curative bias, 35; and diagnosis, 21-22, 68, 85; and dualism, 5, 6, 33-38, 98; and doctor-patient relationship, 78-79, 121, 128-129; and empiricism, 16, 20-21, 54-56, 59-62, 105; and foundationalism, 100; and germ theory, 61-62; ideology of, 4, 8, 34-35, 99; as a language game, 101, 140; and long-term care, 83; and the material body, 17-18, 33, 36, 47, 56-57, 64, 73, 104-105; and mechanistic analogy, 13-14, 38-42, 64; and medical education, 66-67; and medical technology, 26-28, 57-59, 68, 112-113; and norms of health, 24-26, 108, 110-111; and physical reductionism, 42-45; and physiological equilibrium, 25-26, 108; and reductionism, 2, 6-7, 60-61, 64, 76, 97, 102, 105; and regimen and control, 47-48, 65-66; and scientific medicine, 6, 44, 49; and scientific world-view, 28-30; and specific etiology, 45;